Chemical Pathology
interpretative pocket book

Chemical Pathology
interpretative pocket book

RN Walmsley
HJ Cain

Clipath Lab Adelaide

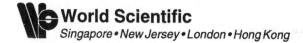

World Scientific
Singapore • New Jersey • London • Hong Kong

Published by

World Scientific Publishing Co. Pte. Ltd.
P O Box 128, Farrer Road, Singapore 912805
USA office: Suite 1B, 1060 Main Street, River Edge, NJ 07661
UK office: 57 Shelton Street, Covent Garden, London WC2H 9HE

British Library Cataloguing-in-Publication Data
A catalogue record for this book is available from the British Library.

CHEMICAL PATHOLOGY: INTERPRETATIVE POCKET BOOK

ISBN   981-02-2802-3
       981-02-2849-X (pbk)

Printed in Singapore.

Preface

This text, designed as a companion volume to *Cases in Chemical Pathology: A diagnostic Approach* (World Scientific, Singapore), contains basic information on interpretative chemical pathology in the form of lists of causes and , where appropriate, information on evaluation in the form of algorithms.

Basically it is devised as a practical guide for medical students, medical practitioners, and clinical chemists. It does not attempt to cover all tests but has concentrated on those tests most frequently used by clinicians and the commonly observed abnormalities.

We make no claim of infallibility in the area of evaluation and interpretation and recognise that others may do these things differently. The information given is based on our experience in teaching hospitals and in providing services to general practitioners.

Adelaide, April 1996

RN Walmsley
HJ Cain

Contents

1 Introduction

The unexpected result:

Consider:
- Artefact *(page 3)*
- Reference range, eg, sex, age
- Laboratory error, eg, analytical interference
- Sampling error, eg, specimen from drip arm
- Labelling error, ie, different patient
- Incorrect sample storage, eg, serum sitting on cells

Appropriate action: Obtain a fresh sample from the patient and re-analyse

Significant change in an analyte value

Consider:

1. Biological variation:
2. Time of day (circadian rhythm)
3. Relation to meals
4. Posture
5. Analytical imprecision *(page 2)**

* The implication is that a given value (x) has a 95% chance of lying within the limits $x \pm 2SD$. For example, a plasma [Na] of 140 mmol/L with an error of 3 mmol/L has a value between 137 and 143 mmol/L. For a significant increase to occur the value has to be 147 mmol/L (144–150 mmol/L)

Laboratory test analytical errors (2SD)

Plasma Analyte	Error		Rule of thumb
Sodium	3	mmol/L	~2.5%
Potassium	0.1	mmol/L	"
Chloride	2	mmol/L	"
Calcium	0.06	mmol/L	"
Urate	0.01	mmol/L	"
Albumin	2	g/L	~5.0%
Phosphate	0.04	mmol/L	"
Free T_4	1.0	pmol/L	"
TSH	0.20	mIU/L	"
ALT, AST	3	U/L	~10%
Amylase	20	U/L	"
ALP	8	U/L	"
CK	5	U/L	"
GGT	3	U/L	"
Cortisol	10	nmol/L	"
Glucose	0.4	mmol/L	"
Urea	0.5	mmol/L	"
HCO_3	2	mmol/L	"
Bilirubin	3	µmol/L	~15%
Creatinine	0.02	mmol/L	"

Some common causes of artefactual results

Plasma Analyte	Effect	Cause
Albumin	*increased*	prolonged application of tourniquet
Bilirubin	*decreased*	prolonged exposure to light
Bicarbonate	*decreased*	prolonged exposure to air
Calcium	*increased*	prolonged application of tourniquet
	decreased	collected into EDTA container
Cortisol	*increased*	prednisone therapy; stress
Creatinine	*increased*	high plasma acetoacetate
Glucose	*increased*	patient not fasting
	decreased	no fluoride preservative
Phosphate	*increased*	prolonged contact with red cells, haemolysis
Potassium	*increased*	prolonged contact with red cells; collected into K_2EDTA container; haemolysis; contamination by IV infusion
Sodium	*increased*	contamination by IV infusion
	decreased	hyperlipidaemia; contamination by IV infusion
Triglyceride	*increased*	patient not fasted
Urine Analyte		
Calcium	*decreased*	no acid preservative in container
Phosphate	*decreased*	no acid preservative in container
Metanephrines	*increased*	drugs (e.g. chlorpromazine)
Porphobilinogen	*decreased*	exposure to light

2 Sodium

Hyponatraemia *(see Figure page 7)*

Commonest causes
- Acute water overload (IV) in post-operative subjects
- Drugs (including diuretics)
- Syndrome of inappropriate secretion of ADH (SIADH)

Eutonic hyponatraemia *(POsmol normal)*
Pseudohyponatraemia: *hyperlipidaemia, hyperproteinaemia*

Hypertonic hyponatraemia *(POsmol high)*
Hyperglycaemia, mannitol, glycine

Hypotonic hyponatraemia *(POsmol low)*

Hypovolaemia
(A) *Extrarenal (U[Na] <20 mmol/L)*
Gastrointestinal loss: *diarrhoea, vomiting*
Skin loss: *excessive sweating*
(B) *Renal (U [Na] >20 mmol/L)*
Diuretic therapy, Salt-losing nephritis, Addison's disease

Euvolaemia
(A) *with U[Na] <20 mmol/L*
(Acute water overload): *Increased water intake PLUS:*
Hypovolaemia: *haemorrhage, burns, drugs (page 5)*
Stress: *post-surgery, psychogenic*
Endocrine: *hypothyroidism, cortisol deficiency*
Renal insufficiency

.... *Cont'd next page*

(Hyponatraemia continued)
(B) *with U[Na] >20 mmol/L*
    (Chronic water overload):
    SIADH *(page 6)*
    Drugs *(page 5)*
    Chronic renal failure
    Endocrine: *hypothyroidism, cortisol deficiency*

Hypervolaemia (Oedematous states)
urine [Na] <20 mmol/L
    Cardiac failure
    Cirrhosis of liver
    Nephrotic syndrome

SIADH Syndrome of inappropriate secretion of antidiuretic hormone.

Drugs associated with hyponatraemia

Increased ADH secretion
    Hypnotics/Narcotics: barbiturates, morphine
    Hypoglycaemics: chlorpropamide, tolbutamide
    Antineoplastics: vincristine, vinblastine, cyclophosphamide
    Anticonvulsants: carbamazepine
    Miscellaneous: clofibrate, isoprenaline, nicotine derivatives

Potentiation of ADH action
    chlorpropamide
    paracetamol
    indomethacin

Diuretics
    thiazides, frusemide, spironolactone, amiloride, triamterene

---

Syndrome of inappropriate secretion of anti-diuretic hormone (SIADH)

Tumours
  Carcinoma: bronchus, prostate, thymus, pancreas
  Brain neoplasms: glioma, meningioma
Brain pathology
  Tumours: glioma, meningioma
  Trauma
  Infection: encephalitis, meningitis, abscess
  Cerebrovascular accident
Pulmonary pathology
  Tumours: carcinoma of bronchus
  Infection: pneumonia, tuberculosis

Criteria for diagnosis of SIADH

1. Decreased plasma osmolality
2. Inappropriately high urinary osmolality (eg, >200 mmol/kg)
3. High urinary [Na] (>30 mmol/L)
4. No evidence of hypovolaemia
5. Normal pituitary, adrenal, cardiac, renal, & liver function
6. Absence of therapeutic agents, including diuretics
7. Increased plasma ADH concentration**
8. Response to water restriction (increasing plasma [Na])

** Not always routinely available and unnecessary if all other criteria
satisfied.

Hyponatraemia

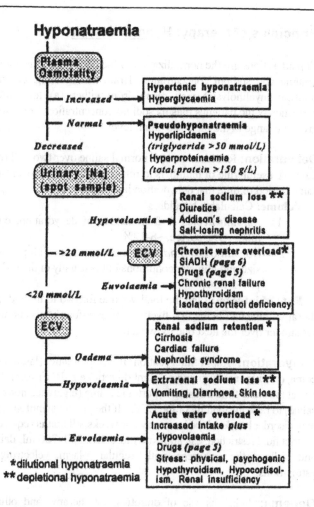

Plasma Osmolality

— *Increased* →

Hypertonic hyponatraemia
Hyperglycaemia

— *Normal* →

Pseudohyponatraemia
Hyperlipidaemia
(triglyceride >50 mmol/L)
Hyperproteinaemia
(total protein >150 g/L)

Decreased

Urinary [Na] (spot sample)

Hypovolaemia →

Renal sodium loss ★★
Diuretics
Addison's disease
Salt-losing nephritis

— >20 mmol/L — **ECV**

Euvolaemia →

Chronic water overload★
SIADH *(page 6)*
Drugs *(page 5)*
Chronic renal failure
Hypothyroidism
Isolated cortisol deficiency

<20 mmol/L

ECV

— *Oedema* →

Renal sodium retention ★
Cirrhosis
Cardiac failure
Nephrotic syndrome

— *Hypovolaemia* →

Extrarenal sodium loss ★★
Vomiting, Diarrhoea, Skin loss

— *Euvolaemia* →

Acute water overload ★
Increased intake *plus*
Hypovolaemia
Drugs *(page 5)*
Stress: physical, psychogenic
Hypothyroidism, Hypocortisolism, Renal insufficiency

★dilutional hyponatraemia
★★depletional hyponatraemia

Evaluation of hyponatraemia

Principles of therapy: <u>Hyponatraemia</u>

Considerations are the normalization of the patient's extracellular volume and sodium concentration. Brain damage (e.g. central pontine myelinolysis) may result from either (a) too rapid correction of the patient's plasma sodium concentration, or (b) too great a change in the plasma sodium level

Dehydration: Rehydration with normal saline over two to three days. A useful 'rule of thumb' is to rehydrate the patient over the same period of time that dehydration has occurred.
   Volume: Calculated by adding
   1. *Amount depleted:* from degree of dehydration, e.g. mild, ~5%; severe, ~8-12%.
   2. *Normal daily fluid requirement:* Varies with patient size and climatic conditions but is usually of the order of 1-2 litres.
   Rate of infusion: Plan the total volume for two to three days therapy ; give half in the first twelve to twenty-four hours and the remainder over the next one to two days.

Euhydration: Rapid intervention if symptomatic (lassitude, coma, convulsions) by giving a potent diuretic (e.g. IV Frusemide) and at the same time infusing hypertonic saline (e.g. twice normal saline) to raise the tonicity of the ECF. If the patient symptomless and disorder has developed over days or weeks, all that is required is strict fluid restriction, e.g. allow no more than 500–750 mL daily and follow the progress with regular plasma electrolyte estimations.

Oedema: Judicious use of diuretics, IV therapy, and other specific therapies (e.g. albumin infusions).

Hypernatraemia

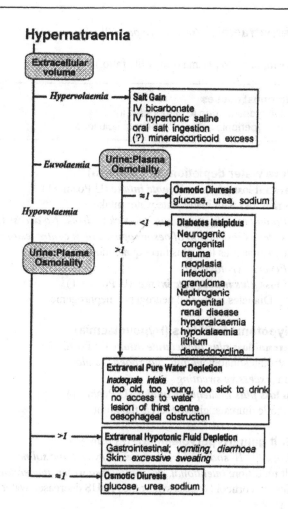

Extracellular volume

— *Hypervolaemia* — **Salt Gain**
IV bicarbonate
IV hypertonic saline
oral salt ingestion
(?) mineralocorticoid excess

— *Euvolaemia* — **Urine:Plasma Osmolality**

≈ 1 → **Osmotic Diuresis**
glucose, urea, sodium

< 1 → **Diabetes Insipidus**
Neurogenic
congenital
trauma
neoplasia
infection
granuloma
Nephrogenic
congenital
renal disease
hypercalcaemia
hypokalaemia
lithium
demeclocycline

Hypovolaemia

Urine:Plasma Osmolality

> 1

Extrarenal Pure Water Depletion
Inadequate intake
too old, too young, too sick to drink
no access to water
lesion of thirst centre
oesophageal obstruction

> 1 → **Extrarenal Hypotonic Fluid Depletion**
Gastrointestinal; *vomiting, diarrhoea*
Skin: *excessive sweating*

≈ 1 → **Osmotic Diuresis**
glucose, urea, sodium

Evaluation of hypernatraemia

Hypernatraemia *(see Figure page 9)*

(U:Posm, urine to plasma osmolality ratio.)

> **Commonest causes**
> ♦ Dehydration due to inadequate intake
> ♦ IV hypertonic saline/bicarbonate solutions

(A) Pure water depletion (Euvolaemia)
Extrarenal loss *plus inadequate intake* (U:Posm >1)
    Normal loss with inadequate water intake:
       Patient too old, too young, too sick to drink; No access to
       water; Obstruction of oesophagus; Thirst centre lesions
    Mucocutaneous loss plus inadequate intake:
       Fever, thyrotoxicosis
Renal loss *plus inadequate intake* (U:Posm <1)
       Diabetes insipidus: neurogenic, nephrogenic

(B) Hypotonic fluid loss (Hypovolaemia)
Extrarenal loss *plus inadequate intake* (U:Posm >1)
    Gastrointestinal: *vomiting, diarrhoea, fistula*
    Skin: *excessive sweating*
Renal loss *plus inadequate intake* (U:Posm ~1)
    Osmotic diuresis: glucose, urea, mannitol

(C) Salt gain (Hypervolaemia) (U:Posm >1)
    Iatrogenic: *IV sodium bicarbonate, IV hypertonic saline*
    Salt ingestion: *intentional, accidental, sea water immersion*
    Mineralocorticoid excess syndromes PLUS decreased water
       intake

Principles of therapy: <u>Hypernatraemia</u>

Pure water depletion (euvolaemia): Water orally if tolerated, or IV infusion of an isotonic solution (5% glucose, 4% glucose in one-fifth normal saline). **Rate:** Estimate the total fluid requirements for two to three days, give half over the first six to twelve hours, and remainder over the next two to three days. The therapy should be constantly monitored by regular plasma electrolyte estimations.

Hypotonic Fluid Depletion (hypovolaemia): Usually significant extracellular volume depletion which may result in peripheral circulatory collapse. Thus first priority is to restore the circulating volume with normal saline. In some situations this may be inadequate and fluids such as blood, plasma, or plasma expanders may be required. Once the plasma volume is restored and the blood pressure returned towards normal, the hypernatraemia is dealt with as outlined above.

Salt Gain (hypervolaemia): If rapid expansion of extracellular volume there is danger of pulmonary oedema and cardiac failure. Remove sodium rapidly using a potent diuretic (e.g. IV frusemide). This will result in a worsening of the hypernatraemia (more water is lost than sodium) and therefore 5% glucose should be infused concurrently.

3 Potassium

Hyperkalaemia *(see Figure page 14)*

> **Commonest causes**
> ♦ Factitious
> ♦ Renal failure
> ♦ Potassium-sparing diuretics
> ♦ Prostaglandin inhibitors, eg NSAIDs

Extrarenal causes
Pseudohyperkalaemia (Factitious)
Haemolysis, Leucocytosis, Thrombocytosis
Increased potassium input
Exogenous: oral/IV therapy
Endogenous: tissue necrosis (crush injury, burns,
malignancy)
Intravascular haemolysis
Disturbed intracellular/extracellular gradient
Acidaemia
Insulin deficiency/diabetes mellitus
Drugs: succinylcholine, digoxin toxicity
Hypertonicity: glucose, sodium
Hyperkalaemic periodic paralysis

Decreased renal potassium excretion
Renal failure
Acute/chronic
Drugs
Diuretics: spironolactone, amiloride, triamterene
Prostaglandin inhibitors: indomethacin, ibuprofen
Others: captopril & other ACE inhibitors, heparin
.... *Cont'd next page*

(Hyperkalaemia continued)
Mineralocorticoid deficient syndromes *(page 46)*
  Hypocortisolism, hypoaldosteronism, high renin:
    Addison's disease, Adrenal C_{21}-hydroxylase defects
  Selective aldosterone deficiency (low renin):
    Syndrome of hyporeninaemic hypoaldosteronism
    Prostaglandin inhibition
  Selective aldosterone deficiency (high renin):
    Heparin therapy;   Corticosterone methyl oxidase deficiency
Mineralocorticoid resistant syndromes *(page 46)*
  High renin and aldosterone:
    Interstitial nephritis; obstructive nephropathy;
    amyloidosis; systemic lupus erythrematosus
    sickle cell disease; pseudohypoaldosteronism

Notes on hyperkalaemia

Severe true hyperkalaemia (eg >7.5 mmol/L) is a medical emergency because of potential effects on the heart (arrhythmia, cardiac arrest) and must be treated promptly regardless of cause. It is not always assocaited with potassium excess, eg, the hyperkalaemia of diabetic ketoacidosis can be associated with a body deficit of 200–400 mmol.

Renal Failure: In uncomplicated *chronic* renal failure hyperkalaemia does not occur until the GFR falls to below 10-20 mL/min (equivalent to a plasma creatinine of >0.40 mmol/L).. In lesser degrees of failure a high potassium suggests a secondary problem, eg high intake, decreased excretion due to drug therapy. In *acute* failure hyper-kalaemia is a consistent feature often occuring early.

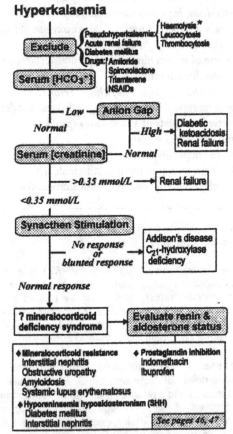

Hyperkalaemia

Exclude
Pseudohyperkalaemia: { Haemolysis*, Leucocytosis, Thrombocytosis }
Acute renal failure
Diabetes mellitus
Drugs: { Amiloride, Spironolactone, Triamterene, NSAIDs }

Serum [HCO₃⁻]

— Low — Anion Gap

Normal

— *High* → Diabetic ketoacidosis, Renal failure

Serum [creatinine] — *Normal*

— >0.35 mmol/L → Renal failure

<0.35 mmol/L

Synacthen Stimulation

No response or blunted response → Addison's disease, C₂₁-hydroxylase deficiency

Normal response

? mineralocorticoid deficiency syndrome

Evaluate renin & aldosterone status

◆ **Mineralocorticoid resistance**
Interstitial nephritis
Obstructive uropathy
Amyloidosis
Systemic lupus erythematosus
◆ **Hyporeninaemia hypoaldosteronism (SHH)**
Diabetes mellitus
Interstitial nephritis

◆ **Prostaglandin inhibition**
Indomethacin
Ibuprofen

See pages 46, 47

* Phosphate and LD may also be increased
Anion Gap = {[Na] + [K]} - {[Cl] + [HCO3]}   RR: 7-17 mEq/L
NSAIDs, non-steroidal anti-inflammatory drugs

Evaluation of hyperkalaemia

Principles of therapy: <u>Hyperkalaemia</u>

For mild elevations of plasma [K], eg <6.0 mmol/L, restriction of intake usually sufficient. Severe elevations may result in cardiac arrhythmias (ventricular fibrillation) and constitute a medical emergency requiring immediate treatment. Therapeutic options include:

Calcium gluconate infusion: 10 to 20 mL as 10% solution given over 2–3 minutes—effect transitory. (Calcium ions antagonize cardiotoxic effects of potassium.) *Note:* Do not add to bicarbonate solutions as calcium carbonate will precipitate in vitro.

Sodium bicarbonate infusion: 100–200 mmol over 30 min. Effective for 2–3 hours. (Metabolic alkalosis forces potassium ions into cells.)

Glucose & insulin infusion: 50 units of soluble insulin infused with 100 mL of 50% glucose—effect lasts several hours. (Insulin stimulates cellular potassium uptake.)

Resonium A (sodium polystyrene sulphonate): Orally or rectally; 30–60 grams twice daily. (Cation exchange resin which binds potassium ions in the gut lumen.)

Haemodialysis: Teatment of choice in acute renal failure or if resistance to above therapies.

Hypokalaemia *(see Figure page 18)*

(*P[HCO$_3$]*, Plasma bicarbonate; *U[K]*, spot urinary potassium; *N*, normal level)

> **Commonest causes**
> ♦ Diuretic therapy
> ♦ Vomiting
> ♦ Diarrhoea
> ♦ Transient

Decreased intake *(P[HCO$_3$]: N, U[K] <20 mmol/L)*
Inadequate IV therapy, Chronic alcoholism, Anorexia nervosa

Transcellular shift *(P[HCO$_3$]: N, U[K]:<20 mmol/L)*
Transient (stress, post carbohydrate meal)
Therapy: insulin, salbutamol, vitamin B$_{12}$
Familial periodic paralysis
Barium toxicity

Extrarenal loss *(P[HCO$_3$]: Low, U[K]: <20 mmol/L)*
Acute diarrhoea, Pancreatic fistula
(P[HCO$_3$]: High, U[K] <20 mmol/L)
Chronic diarrhoea, Laxative abuse, Previous diuretic therapy,
Villous adenoma of colon

Renal loss *(P[HCO$_3$]: Low, U[K] >20 mmol/L)*
Respiratory alkalosis
Renal tubular acidosis
Ureteral diversions .... *Cont'd next page*

(Renal loss continued)
(P[HCO₃]: High, U[K] >20 mmol/L)

    Current diuretic therapy

    Mineralocorticoid excess *(see page 48)*

    Metabolic alkalosis: vomiting, chloride diarrhoea

Bartter's syndrome; Gitelman's syndrome; Liddel's syndrome

Miscellaneous

    Gentamicin (& other aminoglycosides) therapy

    Leukaemia

    Osmotic diuresis

    Post-obstructive nephropathy

    Post-acute tubular necrosis

    Magnesium depletion

Notes on hypokalaemia

Transient: Mild hypokalaemia, of no obvious cause, which corrects itself without specific therapy. Often assocaited with acute illness and stress related disorders — probably due to stimulation of β-receptors by stress-produced catecholamines.

Magnesium depletion: Consider this condition (Table on page 65) if hypokalaemia is resistant to potassium therapy or if there is a coexisting hypocalcaemia. Common in chronic alcoholics.

Urinary [K]: Always take a spot urine for this estimation before commencing potassium therapy, oral or IV — up to 50% of administered potassium appears in the urine within 2 to 4 hours.

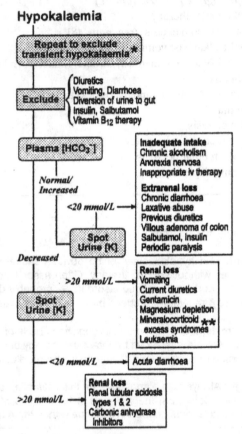

Hypokalaemia

Repeat to exclude transient hypokalaemia*

Exclude
- Diuretics
- Vomiting, Diarrhoea
- Diversion of urine to gut
- Insulin, Salbutamol
- Vitamin B_{12} therapy

Plasma [HCO_3^-]

Inadequate intake
Chronic alcoholism
Anorexia nervosa
Inappropriate iv therapy

Normal/Increased

Extrarenal loss
Chronic diarrhoea
Laxative abuse
Previous diuretics
Villous adenoma of colon
Salbutamol, insulin
Periodic paralysis

<20 mmol/L ⟶ **Spot Urine [K]**

Decreased

>20 mmol/L ⟶ **Renal loss**
Vomiting
Current diuretics
Gentamicin
Magnesium depletion
Mineralocorticoid **
  excess syndromes
Leukaemia

Spot Urine [K]

<20 mmol/L ⟶ Acute diarrhoea

>20 mmol/L ⟶ **Renal loss**
Renal tubular acidosis
  types 1 & 2
Carbonic anhydrase
  inhibitors

*Transient hypokalaemia: adrenergic (stress), post-carbohydrate meals, post-exercise

** *See pages 48, 49*

Evaluation of hypokalaemia

Principles of therapy: Hypokalaemia

Three points to consider:

- Potassium deficient subjects who are hypokalaemic are usually at least 200 mmols depleted
- Average daily intake is 100 mmol & 1 g of KCl contains 14 mmol of K
- Up to 50% of administered K (oral & IV) is lost in urine within 2–4 hours

Oral therapy: Choice for moderate degrees of hypokalaemia (eg >2.5 mmol/L). Most effective is effervescent potassium (eg Chlorvescent, ~14 mmol of K/tablet). **NB** One Slow-K table given three-times daily equals 24 mmol of K (equivalent to giving ~12 mmol/day as 50% lost in urine).

Intravenous therapy: Give KCl infusion in severe hypokalaemia (eg plasma K <2.0 mmol/L). Usual preparationis a 10 mL ampule of 10% KCl (1g of KCl or ~14 mmol of K per ampule). To prevent development of severe hyperkalaemia give as follows:

- At concentration <40 mmol/L (not more than 3 g KCl/L of carrier fluid)
- At rate <20 mmol/hour
- Regular monitoring of plasma K, particularly if any degree of renal insufficiency

Note As subject becomes potassium replete, eg plasma [K] & [HCO_3]nearing normal values, slow the infusion as a stage is soon reached when a small amount of infused K will produce a disproportionate rise in the plasma level (over-shoot).

4 Acid-base

Metabolic acidosis   *(see Figure page 23)*

Commonest causes	Primary lesion
♦ Renal insufficiency	Fall in Plasma $[HCO_3]$
♦ Diarrhoea	**Types**
♦ Lactic acidosis	High anion gap
♦ Diabetic ketoacidosis	Normal anion gap

Plasma Anion Gap:
{ [Na] mmol/L + [K] mmol/L} − { [HCO₃] mmol/L + [Cl]}

High anion gap metabolic acidosis

Renal failure: acute, chronic
Ketoacidosis: diabetic, alcoholic, starvation
Lactic acidosis (page 21)
Toxins: ethanol, methanol, paraldehyde, salicylate,
     ethylene glycol

Normal anion gap metabolic acidosis

Hyperkalaemic
Early uraemic acidosis
Obstructive uropathy
Renal tubular acidosis Type 4: mineralocorticoid
     deficiency, tubule unresponsiveness   *(page 45)*
Ingestions/infusions: HCl, lysine/arginine-HCl,
     ammonium chloride
Diabetic ketoacidosis: post-therapy

.... *Cont'd next page*

(Metabolic acidosis continued)
Hypokalaemic
Diarrhoea
Renal tubular acidosis: Type 1, Type 2 *(pages 43, 44)*
Carbonic anhydrase inhibition: acetazolamide
Urinary diversions: ureterosigmoidostomy, vesico-colic
   fistula, obstructed ileal bladder
Post-hypocapnic acidosis

Lactic acidosis

> **Commonest causes**
> ♦ Shock/hypovolaemia
> ♦ Convulsions/severe exercise
> ♦ Diabetes mellitus

L-lactic acidosis

Type A (tissue hypoxia apparent)
   Hypoxia, severe anaemia, shock, congestive cardiac failure
Type B (tissue hypoxia not apparent)
   Acquired disease: diabetes mellitus, liver failure, convulsions,
      tumours
   Drugs/toxins: biguanides, ethanol, methanol
   Congenital disorders: glucose-6-phosphatase deficiency,
      fructose-1,6-bisphosphatase deficiency
Toxins
   Salicylate, ethanol, methanol, paraldehyde, ethylene glycol
D-lactic acidosis
   Short bowel syndrome

Principlesof treatment: <u>Metabolic Acidosis</u>

Aim is to increase the extracellular bicarbonate concentration by (a) treating the primary disorder, or (b) bicarbonate therapy.

Parenteral bicarbonate therapy

Indications. Consider if blood pH below 7.20; necessary in RTA (Types 1 & 2) and should be considered in severe acidaemia associated with diarrhoea. *If considering bicarbonate therapy it is important that the **patient's potassium status be normalised** prior to administration as existent hypokalaemia will worsen due to cellular uptake.*

Aim. Raise the pH above 7.20 or the plasma [HCO_3] to 15–20 mmol/L.

Amount: Calculated from the patient's body weight and the plasma [HCO_3] — assume 'bicarbonate space' to be 50% of body weight, eg to raise [HCO_3] by 10 mmol/L in a 70-kg patient would require: 0.5 x 70 x 10 = 350 mmol. In practice the patient is usually 'titrated' by slowly infusing bicarbonate and regularly checking the plasma [HCO_3].

Complications: (a) *sodium overload*; (b) *hypokalaemia*; (c) *tetany* — alkalaemia enhances the binding of Ca^{++} to protein; (d) *'overshoot' alkalosis* — particularly if organic anions (lactate, ketones) are present (converted to bicarbonate when metabolised).

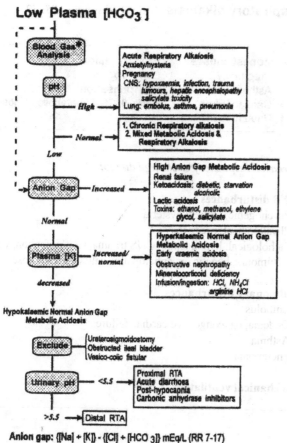

Low Plasma [HCO₃]

Blood Gas Analysis

Acute Respiratory Alkalosis
Anxiety/hysteria
Pregnancy
CNS: *hypoxaemia, infection, trauma*
tumours, hepatic encephalopathy
salicylate toxicity
Lung: *embolus, asthma, pneumonia*

pH — *High*

— *Normal* →
1. Chronic Respiratory alkalosis
2. Mixed Metabolic Acidosis &
   Respiratory Alkalosis

Low

Anion Gap — *Increased* →
High Anion Gap Metabolic Acidosis
Renal failure
Ketoacidosis: *diabetic, starvation*
alcoholic
Lactic acidosis
Toxins: *ethanol, methanol, ethylene*
glycol, salicylate

Normal

Plasma [K] — *Increased/ normal* →
Hyperkalaemic Normal Anion Gap
Metabolic Acidosis
Early uraemic acidosis
Obstructive nephropathy
Mineralocorticoid deficiency
Infusion/ingestion: *HCl, NH₄Cl*
arginine HCl

decreased

Hypokalaemic Normal Anion Gap
Metabolic Acidosis

Exclude
Ureterosigmoidostomy
Obstructed ileal bladder
Vesico-colic fistular

Urinary pH — <5.5 →
Proximal RTA
Acute diarrhoea
Post-hypocapnia
Carbonic anhydrase inhibitors

>5.5 → Distal RTA

Anion gap: {[Na] + [K]} - {[Cl] + [HCO₃]} mEq/L (RR 7-17)

RTA: Renal Tubular Acidosis

* If blood gases unavailable exclude respiratory alkalosis on clinical grounds

Evaluation of a low plasma bicarbonate

Respiratory alkalosis *(see Figures pages 23, 32)*

Commonest causes	Primary lesion
♦ Pregnancy	Low P_{CO_2}
♦ Asthma	**Compensation**
♦ Cardiac failure	Fall in $[HCO_3]$ (metabolic acidosis)
♦ Pneumonia	

Increased respiratory exchange due to:

CNS disturbances
Psychogenic: anxiety/hysteria
Physiological: pregnancy
Pathological: hypoxaemia, CNS trauma, CNS infection, CNS
tumours, hepatic encephalopathy, salicylate overdose

Pulmonary disturbances
Embolus
Oedema, eg, congestive cardiac failure
Asthma
Pneumonia

Mechanical ventilation

Metabolic alkalosis *(see Figure page 27)*

Commonest causes	Primary lesion
♦ Diuretic therapy	Rise in plasma [HCO$_3$]
♦ Vomiting	**Types**
♦ Mineralocorticoid excess syndromes *(page 48)*	(1) Respond to saline infusion – *saline responsive*
	(2) No response to infusion – *saline unresponsive*

(A) Saline responsive (ECV contraction, *Urine [Cl] <20 mmol/L)*

Gastrointestinal H$^+$ loss: vomiting, gastric suction,
Renal H$^+$ loss: diuretic therapy: current*, previous; post-hypercapnia
Exogenous load: bicarbonate (IV, oral), antacids (magnesium carbonate), organic acid salts (lactate, citrate, acetate)
Contraction alkalosis

(B) Saline unresponsive (ECV expansion, *Urine [Cl] >20 mmol/L)*

Mineralocorticoid excess: primary hyperaldosteronism, Bartter's syndrome, Liddle's syndrome, liquorice ingestion, carbenoxolone therapy
Cortisol and mineralocorticoid excess: Cushing's syndrome, ectopic ACTH syndrome, enzyme defects (C$_{11}$ & C$_{17}$-hydroxylase deficiency), severe potassium depletion

Note: *Current diuretic therapy will have a urine [Cl] >20 mmol/L.

Principles of treatment: <u>Metabolic Alkalosis</u>

Depends on the cause and severity, the aim being to lower the plasma [HCO_3] (by removing both generating and maintenance mechanisms).

In the *volume-contracted (saline-responsive)* group, the hypovolaemia is treated by IV saline and the potassium deficiency, by the appropriate therapy (page 8). The *saline-unresponsive metabolic alkalosis* due to mineralocorticoid excess should be managed by removing the source of the mineralocorticoid, if possible, and correcting the potassium deficiency. Interim treatment can be carried out by administering spironolactone or amiloride which (a) decreases the extracellular volume (diuretic), and (b) prevents renal potassium wasting.

In the rare severe case where the alkalosis is *symptomatic* (twitching and tetany) and rapid intervention is required, acetazolamide may be used to increase the renal excretion of bicarbonate. In life-threatening cases treatment with HCl infusions and cimetidine may be necessary.

High plasma [HCO₃⁻]

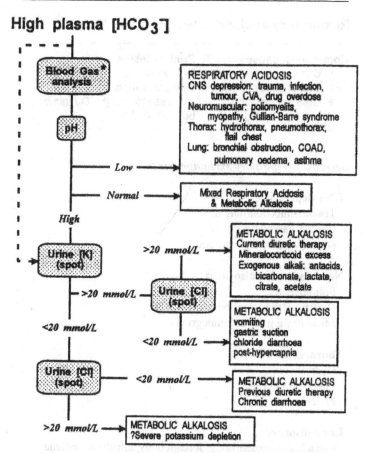

RESPIRATORY ACIDOSIS
CNS depression: trauma, infection,
    tumour, CVA, drug overdose
Neuromuscular: poliomyelits,
    myopathy, Gullian-Barre syndrome
Thorax: hydrothorax, pneumothorax,
    flail chest
Lung: bronchial obstruction, COAD,
    pulmonary oedema, asthma

Mixed Respiratory Acidosis
& Metabolic Alkalosis

METABOLIC ALKALOSIS
Current diuretic therapy
Mineralocorticoid excess
Exogenous alkali: antacids,
    bicarbonate, lactate,
    citrate, acetate

METABOLIC ALKALOSIS
vomiting
gastric suction
chloride diarrhoea
post-hypercapnia

METABOLIC ALKALOSIS
Previous diuretic therapy
Chronic diarrhoea

METABOLIC ALKALOSIS
?Severe potassium depletion

* If blood gases not available exclude respiratory acidosis on
clinical grounds and perform spot urinary [K] & [Cl] estimations.

Evaluation of a high plasma bicarbonate

Respiratory acidosis *(see Figures page 27, 31)*

Commonest causes	Primary lesion
♦ Chronic lung disease	High P_{CO_2}
♦ Bronchial obstruction	**Compensation**
♦ CNS depression	Increased plasma $[HCO_3]$ (metabolic alkalosis)

Decreased respiratory exchange due to:

CNS depression
Trauma/infection/tumour
Cerebrovascular accident
Drug overdose e.g. narcotics

Neuromuscular disorders
Poliomyelitis
Guillain-Barre' syndrome
Myopathy e.g. myasthenia gravis

Thoracic disorders
Hydrothorax
Pneumothorax
Flail chest

Lung disorders
Bronchial obstruction e.g. foreign body, infections, asthma
Emphysema (chronic obstructive airway disease, COAD)
Severe pulmonary oedema

Mechanical ventilation

Evaluation of blood Gases

A set of results should be interpreted as follows:

(1) *Determine status of [H⁺]*

pH: >7.45 — alkalaemia
     <7.35 — acidaemia
     7.35-7.45 — no disturbance or mixed
                 disturbance

(2) *Determine metabolic component*

[HCO₃]: >33 mmol/L, — metabolic alkalosis
         <23 mmol/L — metabolic acidosis

(3) *Determine respiratory component*

Pco_2: >45 mmHg — respiratory acidosis
          <35 mmHg — respiratory alkalosis

(4) *Combine the information* from (1), (2), and (3). If the patient is acidaemic the primary lesion will be an acidosis (respiratory, metabolic); if the patient is alkalaemic the primary lesion will be a alkalosis (respiratory, metabolic); if the pH is 'normal' (7.35-7.45) consider a mixed disturbance, eg, respiratory acidosis and metabolic alkalosis (page 34).

(5) *Determine if the compensatory response is appropriate* from equations on page 30. If inappropriate consider (a) duration of disorder (i.e., has not had time to compensate), (b) mixed acid-base disorder. The common causes of mixed disorders are on page 34.

Simple acid-base disturbances: characteristics of compensation

Primary disorder	Basic lesion	Compensation	Compensation limits	Final value of compensation
Metabolic Acidosis	$\downarrow[HCO_3]$	$\downarrow Pco_2$	Pco_2: 10 mmHg	Pco_2 mmHg = $1.5\times[HCO_3]+8$ (±2)[1]
Metabolic Alkalosis	$\uparrow[HCO_3]$	$\uparrow Pco_2$	Pco_2: 60 mmHg	Pco_2 mmHg = $0.9\times[HCO_3]+9$ (±2)[2]
Respiratory Acidosis				
Acute	$\uparrow Pco_2$	$\uparrow[HCO_3]$	$[HCO_3]$: ~30mmol/L	$[HCO_3]$: $\uparrow$ by 2-4 mmol/L
Chronic	$\uparrow Pco_2$	$\uparrow[HCO_3]$	$[HCO_3]$: ~45mmol/L	$[HCO_3]$ mmol/L = $0.44\times Pco_2+7.6$[3]
Respiratory Alkalosis				
Acute	$\downarrow Pco_2$	$\downarrow[HCO_3]$	$[HCO_3]$: ~18mmol/L	$[HCO_3]$: $\downarrow$ by 2-4 mmol/L
Chronic	$\downarrow Pco_2$	$\downarrow[HCO_3]$	$[HCO_3]$: ~12mmol/L	May fully compensate (pH ~7.40)

1. Albert MS, et al. *Ann Intern Med* 1967;66:312-322.   2. Fulop M. *NY State J Med* 1976;76:19-23.
3. Engel K, et al. *J App Physiol* 1968;24:288-295

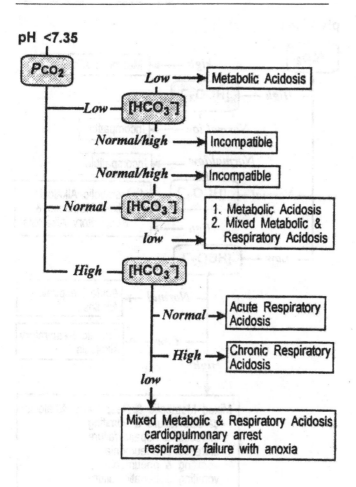

pH <7.35

Pco₂

Low → [HCO₃⁻] → Low → Metabolic Acidosis

Normal/high → Incompatible

Normal → [HCO₃⁻] → Normal/high → Incompatible

low → 1. Metabolic Acidosis
2. Mixed Metabolic & Respiratory Acidosis

High → [HCO₃⁻]

Normal → Acute Respiratory Acidosis

High → Chronic Respiratory Acidosis

low → Mixed Metabolic & Respiratory Acidosis
cardiopulmonary arrest
respiratory failure with anoxia

Blood gas evaluation: Acidaemia

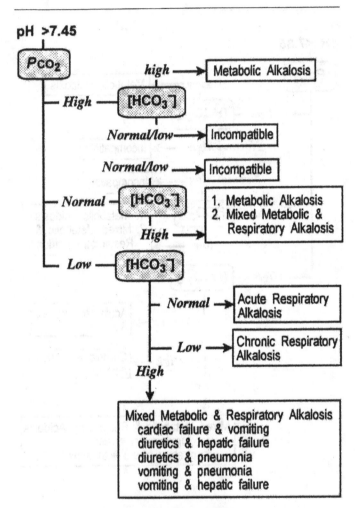

Blood gas evaluation: Alkalaemia

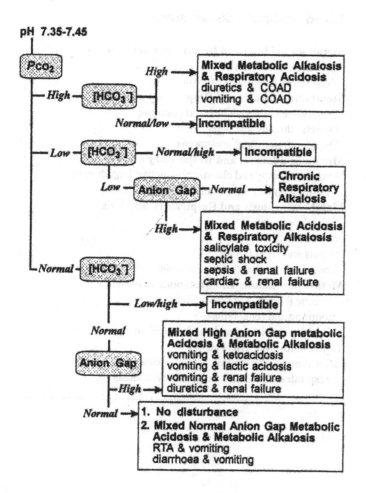

pH 7.35-7.45

Blood gas evaluation: Normal pH

Mixed acid-base disturbances

Metabolic acidosis and Respiratory acidosis
  Cardiopulmonary arrest
  Respiratory failure with anoxia
Metabolic alkalosis and Respiratory alkalosis
  Congestive cardiac failure and vomiting
  Diuretic therapy and hepatic failure
  Diuretic therapy and pneumonia
Metabolic alkalosis and Respiratory acidosis
  Diuretic therapy and chronic obstructive lung disease
  Vomiting and chronic obstructive lung disease
Metabolic acidosis and Respiratory alkalosis
  Salicylate overdose
  Septic shock
  Sepsis and renal failure
  Congestive cardiac failure and renal failure
Metabolic alkalosis and Metabolic acidosis
  Diuretic therapy and ketoacidosis
  Vomiting and renal failure
  Vomiting and lactic acidosis/ketoacidosis
Triple acid-base disturbance
  Mixed metabolic acidosis and alkalosis PLUS
    respiratory alkalosis or respiratory acidosis

5 Renal disease

Plasma Urea & Creatinine: Increased

Commonest causes
- ♦ Decreased GFR

Analytical interference & increased production are uncommon but are important in that may give a misleading impression about the subject's renal function.

Decreased GFR (Creatinine & Urea)

Pre-renal: shock/haemorrhage, dehydration, congestive cardiac failure
Renal: acute and chronic renal failure
Post-renal: obstructive lesions of the urinary tract

Analytical interference (Creatinine only)

Ketosis: acetoacetate
Drugs: cephalosporins, e.g. cefoxitin

Increased production

Creatinine: dietary (roasted meats especially game), Large muscle mass
Urea: High protein meal*, Haemorrhage to gut *

* Plasma urea elevated only if associated depressed GFR

Chronic renal failure: Causes

Definition
Progressive azotaemia — elevated plasma urea & creatinine concentrations — due to a falling glomerular filtration rate (GFR) occurring over weeks, months, or years.

Diabetic nephropathy	33%
Hypertensive nephrosclerosis	29%
Glomerulonephritis	15%
Tubulointerstitial	6%
Obstructive nephropathy	
Analgesic nephropathy	
Congenital disorders	5%
Polycystic kidney	
Medullary cystic disease	

Degree of renal insufficiency and appearance of abnormal plasma analyte levels in progressive chronic renal failure. Creat Clr, Creatinine clearance.

Plasma [Creat] (mmol/L)	Creat Clr (mL/min)	Raised analyte
<0.12	90-120	nil
0.20	30-60	urea, creatinine
0.30	20-30	K^+, H^+, anion gap
0.40	10-20	phosphate, urate (hypocalcaemia)

Acute renal failure: Causes

> **Definition**
>
> Sudden increase in plasma urea and creatinine (azotaemia) due to a decrease in the GFR occuring over hours or days.
>
> The decline in GFR may be due to:
> (1)   Reduced renal blood perfusion: ***prerenal uraemia***, functional impairment
> (2)   Parenchymal renal disease: renal uraemia, ***acute tubular necrosis***
> (3)   Urinary tract obstruction: ***postrenal uraemia***

Prerenal failure

Dehydration
Shock/Trauma/Surgery
Haemorrhage
Cardiac failure

Parenchymal renal disease ('Acute renal failure')

Acute tubular necrosis: *Ischaemic, Nephrotoxic*
Interstitial nephritis: *Infection, Drug hypersensitivity*
Acute glomerulonephritis
Renal artery occlusion (bilateral)
Thrombotic microangiopathy: *Thrombocytopenic purpura,*
    Haemolytic uraemic syndrome, Malignant hypertension
Cortical necrosis: *Gram-negative sepsis, Obstetrical accidents.*

.... *Cont'd next page*

(Acute renal failure continued)

Postrenal failure

Ureteral obstruction: *Stones, Clots, Papillary necrosis, urate crystals, External pressure*

Bladder neck obstruction: *Prostatic hypertrophy, Malignancy, Calculi, Functional Neuropathy*

Urethral obstruction: *Stones, Stricture*

Differentation between prerenal failure (PRU) & acute tubular necrosis (ATN):

Most useful single test is inspection of urinary sediment:
  PRU: Clear
  ATN: Blood, Cells, Casts
The biochemical indices shown below are useful but may be misleading.

Urinary electrolytes and derived indices in prerenal uraemia and acute tubular necrosis (ATN).

Index/units	Prerenal uraemia	ATN
Urine osmol (mmol/kg)	>500	<350
Urine [Na] (mmol/L)	<20	>40
FENa (%)*	<1	>3
U:P[Creat]	>40	<20

* Fractional excretion of sodium

$$FE_{Na} (\%) = \frac{UNa}{PNa} \times \frac{PCr}{Ucr} \times 100$$

(UNa=urinary [Na], PNa=plasma [Na], PCr=plasma [creatinine], UCr=urinary [creatinine])

Nephrotic syndrome

Characteristics & Diagnosis
  Oedema
  Proteinuria: >3 g/24h
  Hypoalbuminaemia: <30 g/L
  Hyperlipidaemia: hypercholesterolaemia
Common causes
  ♦ 90% of all cases are in children (idiopathic)
      70% Minimal change
      20% Proliferative/membranoproliferative
          glomerulonephritis
      5%–10% Focal glomerulosclerosis
  ♦ 10% of all cases are in adults
      30%–40% Secondary (mainly diabetes mellitus)
      70% Idiopathic

Primary (idiopathic)
  Minimal change disease
  Membranous nephropathy
  Proliferative glomerulonephritis
  Membranoproliferative glomerulonephritis
  Focal glomerulosclerosis
  IgA nephropathy
Secondary
  Diabetes mellitus
  Amyloidosis
  Collagen disease (SLE, polyarthritis, Sjogren's syndrome)
  Malignancy (myeloma, lymphoma)
  Infections (poststreptococcal, endocarditis, hepatitis, malaria)
  Heavy metal toxicity
  Drugs (probenecid, penicillamine, gold, captopril)
  Hereditary (Alport's syndrome, Congenital)

Proteinuria   *(>0.50 g/day)*

Glomerular (Albumin 90-99%)
Isolated (<1–2 g/day)
　　Functional: *fever, severe exercise, cardiac failure, stress*
　　Orthostatic
　　Transient benign
　　Intermittent benign
Renal disease (1–5 g/day)
　　Nephrotic syndrome
　　Glomerulonephritis
　　Tubulointerstitial disease

Tubular (<2 g/day, Albumin 10–20%)
　　Fanconi syndrome

Overflow (small MW proteins, no albuminuria)
　　Dysgammaglobulinaemias, e.g. myeloma

Secretory (mucoproteins, IgA)
　　Inflammatory processes of urinary passages

Type: The protein species in the urine differs in the four types of proteinuria.

Glomerular:　mainly albumin (90-99%)
Tubular:　mainly α- and β-globulins (e.g. β_2-micro-globulins), albumin 10-20%
Overflow:　free light chains of monoclonal IgG, IgA, or IgD, haemoglobin, myoglobin
Secretory: mucoproteins, secretory IgA

Renal acidosis *(see Figure p. 42, Table p. 43)*

(1) High anion gap

Renal failure: acute, chronic

(2) Normal anion gap (hyperchloraemic)

Hyperkalaemia
    'early' uraemic acidosis
    Obstructive uropathy
    Mineralocorticoid deficient syndromes (Type 4 RTA):
        decreased aldosterone production (page 46)
        tubular unresponsiveness (page 46)
    Hyperkalaemic distal renal tubular acidosis:
    Obstructive nephropathy
    Sickle cell disease of kidney

Hypokalaemia
    Renal tubular acidosis:
        Type 1 (distal RTA, page 44)
        Type 2 (proximal RTA, page 45)
        Type 3 (Type 1 with bicarbonate wasting)

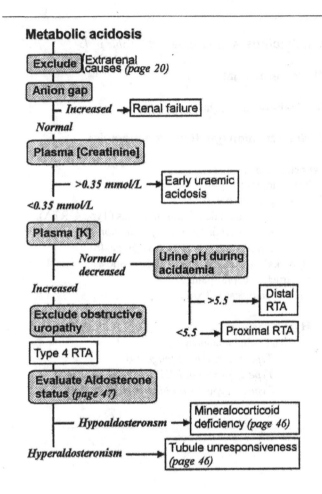

Evaluation of renal acidosis

Laboratory diagnosis of the renal acidoses.

	Plasma [K]	Plasma [Creat]	UpH during acidosis*	UTA during acidosis* (mmol/min)	UNH$_4$ during acidosis* (mmol/min)	Urinary FE$_{HCO3}$** (%)
Normal	N	N	4.6-5.3	24-51	33-75	<1
Type 1	N-D	N-sl I	>5.5	<24	<33	<3
Type 2	N-D	N-sl I	<5.5	>24	>33	>15
Type 3	N-D	N-sl I	>5.5	<24	<33	5-10
Type 4	I	N-sl I	<5.5	<24	<33	5-10
Uraemic	N-I	I++	<5.5	<25	<35	<5-30

U urine, N normal, D decreased, I increased, sl I slightly increased, I$^+$ greatly increased, UTA urine titratable acidity, UNH$_4$ urine ammonia, FE$_{HCO3}$ fractional excretion of bicarbonate

* patient should be acidaemic (pH <7.35 or HCO$_3$ <16 mmol/L)
** patient should have a normal plasma [bicarbonate]

Renal tubular acidosis - Type 1 (distal)

Defect in renal tubular hydrogen ion secretion

Primary
   Sporadic
   Hereditary

Secondary
Autoimmune disorders: Sjogrens syndrome, primary
   biliary cirrhosis, chronic active hepatitis,
   dysgammaglobulinaemia

Nephrocalcinosis: idiopathic hypercalciuria, primary
   hyperparathyroidism, vitamin D intoxication,
   medullary sponge disease

Inborn errors of metabolism: Wilson's disease, Fabry's
   disease, Ehlers-Danlos syndrome, sickle cell anaemia,
   Marfan's syndrome

Toxins/drugs: amphotericin B, lithium, analgesics,
   toluene

Renal disease: pyelonephritis, obstructive uropathy,
   renal transplant, analgesic nephropathy

Renal tubular acidosis - Type 2 (proximal)

Defect in renal bicarbonate reabsorption

Primary

Sporadic
Hereditary

Secondary

Inborn errors of metabolism: cystinosis, Lowe's
syndrome, Wilson's disease, tyrosinaemia

Drugs/toxins: out of date tetracyclines, lead, carbonic anhydrase
inhibitors

Renal disease: amyloidosis, nephrotic syndrome, renal
transplant, medullary cystic disease, multiple
myeloma

Secondary hyperparathyroidism: vitamin D deficiency

6 Mineralocorticoids

Mineralocorticoid deficiency *(see Figure page 47)*

The features of mineralocorticoid deficiency include:

♦ *Hyperkalaemia:* decreased renal potassium excretion
♦ *Hyponatraemia and hypovolaemia:* decreased renal sodium reabsorption
♦ *Normal anion gap metabolic acidosis:* reduced net renal hydrogen ion (H^+) excretion

---

Drugs
Potassium-sparing diuretics: *amiloride, spironolactone, triamterene*
Prostaglandin inhibitors: *indomethacin, ibuprofen*
Miscellaneous: *heparin, Captopril*

Deficient cortisol and aldosterone
Addison's disease; C_{21}-hydroxylase deficiency

Deficient aldosterone and normal cortisol
Syndrome of hyporeninaemic hypoaldosteronism: *diabetes mellitus, interstitial nephritis, prostaglandin inhibitors*
Enzyme defects: *corticosterone methyl oxidase (CMO) deficiency*

Tubular unresponsiveness *(increased aldosterone and renin)*
Renal disease: *interstitial nephritis, obstructive nephropathy, amyloidosis, systemic lupus erythematosus (SLE)*
Renal transplant
Pseudohypoaldosteronism
Chloride shunt

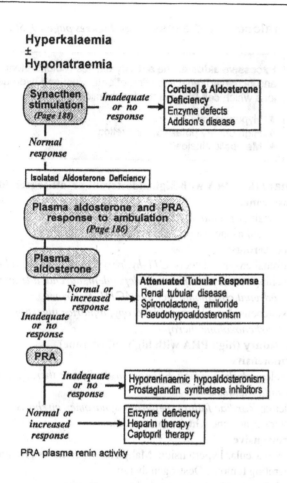

Evaluation of (?) mineralocorticoid deficiency

Mineralocorticoid excess *(see Figures page 49, 50)*

> **Excessive aldosterone activity** causes sodium retention and increased renal excretion of potassium and hydrogen ions which can result in the biochemical picture of
>
> ♦ Hypokalaemia
> ♦ High urinary potassium excretion
> ♦ Metabolic alkalosis.

Primary (low PRA with high aldosterone or other steroids)
Aldosterone:
    Adrenal: *adenoma, hyperplasia, carcinoma*
    Dexamethasone-suppressible hyperaldosteronism
Other steroids:
    Adrenal enzyme defects: *C11-hydroxylase, C17-hydroxylase*
    Cushing's syndrome: *pituitary dependent, adrenal adenoma,*
        adrenal carcinoma, ectopic ACTH syndrome
    Exogenous steroids: *steroid therapy, liquorice ingestion,*
        carbenoxolone therapy
Secondary (high PRA with high aldosterone)
Normotensive:
    Physiological: *dehydration, haemorrhage, diuretic therapy, renal*
        tubular acidosis
    Oedema: *cardiac failure, nephrotic syndrome, cirrhosis*
    Bartter's syndrome; Gitelman's syndrome
Hypertensive:
    Renovascular hypertension; Malignant hypertension; Renin-
    secreting tumour; Oestrogen therapy
Pseudohyperaldosteronism (Liddle's syndrome)

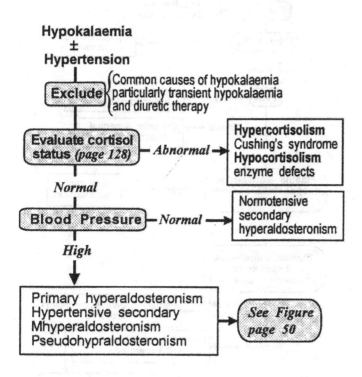

Hypokalaemia
±
Hypertension

Exclude { Common causes of hypokalaemia particularly transient hypokalaemia and diuretic therapy

Evaluate cortisol status *(page 128)* — *Abnormal* → **Hypercortisolism** Cushing's syndrome **Hypocortisolism** enzyme defects

Normal

Blood Pressure — *Normal* → Normotensive secondary hyperaldosteronism

High

Primary hyperaldosteronism
Hypertensive secondary
Mhyperaldosteronism
Pseudohypraldosteronism → *See Figure page 50*

Evaluation of (?) mineralocorticoid excess

HYPERTENSION
+
PLASMA [K] < 4.0 mmol/L

Exclude — {diuretic therapy
              {Cushing's syndrome

Urinary [K] — *<20 mmol/L* → Hyperaldosteronism unlikely

>20 mmol/L

PRA — *High* → Hypertensive secondary hyperaldosteronism

— *Normal* → Consider essential hypertension

Low

Plasma aldosterone response to sodium load *(page 187)* — *Suppression* → Low renin hypertension

No suppression

Plasma aldosterone response to ambulation *(page 186)*

No change or fall → Primary hyperaldosteronism ? adenoma

Increase → Primary hyperaldosteronism ? hyperplasia

Diagnostic imaging Adrenal vein sampling

(PRA plasma renin activity)

Evaluation of (?) primary hyperaldosteronism

7 Calcium

Hypercalcaemia *(see Figure page 53)*

> **Commonest causes** *(exclude hyperalbuminaemia)*
> ♦ Primary hyperparathyroidism
> ♦ Malignancy
> ♦ Vitamin D excess

Malignancy
Solid neoplasms: *breast, bronchus, bone, cervix, ovary, gut, kidney, pancreas, liver, testicle, thyroid, prostate, melanoma*
Haematological: *multiple myeloma, Waldenstrom's macro-globulinaemia, non-Hodgkin's lymphoma, Hodgkin's disease, leukaemia*

Hyperparathyroidism
Primary hyperparathyroidism, Tertiary hyperparathyroidism, Multiple endocrine neoplasia

Non-malignant/non-parathyroid causes
Hyperalbuminaemia: *dehydration, prolonged tourniquet application*
Increased intake/absorption: *vitamin D excess, sarcoidosis, milk-alkali syndrome, IV infusion*
Increased bone resorption: *thyrotoxicosis, immobilization*
Renal failure: *post-dialysis, post-acute renal failure*
Increased renal reabsorption: *thiazide diuretics, familial hypocalciuric hypercalcaemia*, lithium therapy*
Miscellaneous: *Addison's disease, myxoedema, acromegaly, vitamin A toxicity, phaeochromocytoma, idiopathic hyper-calcaemia of infancy, AIDs*

*Familial benign hypercalcaemia

Hypercalcaemia — Notes on evaluation

The commonest causes are
- Transient
- Primary hyperparathyroidism (PHPT)
- Malignancy
- Vitamin D excess syndromes

Transient: On first testing ~4% of all subjects will have a [Ca] >2.60 mmol/L; on re-testing 75% of these will show normal values (reflects variables such as biological variation, analytical error, etc).

PHPT: Prevalence of ~1:1000; serum ALP & PO_4 values usually normal (abnormalities are late effects of PHPT) Diagnosis confirmed by estimating serum PTH where values >4.0 pmol/L (RR 1.5-6.5) in presence of [Ca] >2.60 mmol/L are indicative of the disorder.

Malignancy: Subject usually known to have tumour. Serum PTH useful to exclude PHPT; values <2.0 pmol/L indicate extra-parathyroid cause for the hypercalcaemia.

Vitamin D excess: Characteristically shows elevation of both [Ca] & [PO_4] & a suppressed serum PTH. Commonest cause is overdosage with calcitriol; other causes are self-medication and sarcoidosis.

Evaluation
1. *Repeat serum [Ca]*, if still elevated then proceed to 2 & 3.
2. *Measure serum PTH*
3. *Estimate urinary calcium excretion rate (UCE):* Usefull test in the young patient as Familial Benign Hypercalcaemia (FBH) is an important cause in these subjects. It is estimated from urinary [Ca] & [Creatinine] (spot urine) & serum [Creatinine] (page 53) the samples being taken simultaneously. In FBH the UCE is low — all other causes of hypercalcaemia have high values.

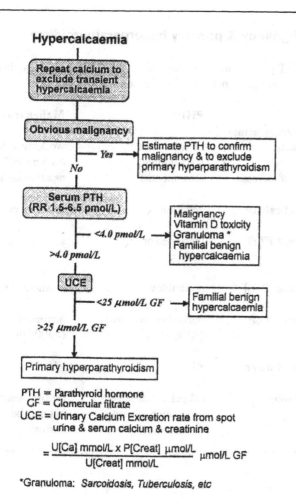

Hypercalcaemia

Repeat calcium to exclude transient hypercalcaemia

Obvious malignancy

Yes → Estimate PTH to confirm malignancy & to exclude primary hyperparathyroidism

No

Serum PTH (RR 1.5-6.5 pmol/L)

<4.0 pmol/L → Malignancy
Vitamin D toxicity
Granuloma *
Familial benign hypercalcaemia

>4.0 pmol/L

UCE

<25 μmol/L GF → Familial benign hypercalcaemia

>25 μmol/L GF

Primary hyperparathyroidism

PTH = Parathyroid hormone
GF = Glomerular filtrate
UCE = Urinary Calcium Excretion rate from spot urine & serum calcium & creatinine

$$= \frac{U[Ca] \text{ mmol/L} \times P[Creat] \text{ } \mu mol/L}{U[Creat] \text{ mmol/L}} \text{ } \mu mol/L \text{ GF}$$

*Granuloma: *Sarcoidosis, Tuberculosis, etc*

Evaluation of hypercalcaemia

Malignancy & primary hyperparathyroidism

(**PHPT** primary hyperparathyroidism **NB** This is a guide only as these findings do not occur in all cases.)

	PHPT	**Malignancy**
Hypercalcaemia		
Duration	months/years	weeks/months
Severity	<3.5 mmol/L	>3.5 mmol/L
Rate of increase	slow:months	rapid:weeks/days
Renal calculi	common	uncommon
Plasma PTH	increased or normal	suppressed
Plasma [PO$_4$]	normal/low	low/normal/high
Plasma ALP	normal or increased (<300 U/L)	increased (>300 U/L)
Urine Ca mmol/d	<10	>10
Radiology	subperiosteal bone resorption, absent lamina dura	osteolytic lesions but may be normal

Hypocalcaemia *(see Figure page 57)*

> **Commonest causes**
> ♦ Hypoalbuminuria
> ♦ Renal failure
> ♦ Acute pancreatitis

Hypoalbuminaemia *(see page 113)*
Vitamin D deficiency
   malnutrition/malabsorption/inadequate TPN
   renal disease
   drugs (phenytoin, barbiturates)
   vitamin D resistance
Hypoparathyroidism
   congenital
   idiopathic
   parathyroid ablation (surgery, infarction)
   magnesium deficiency
   pseudohypoparathyroidism
Increased bone uptake ('hungry bone syndrome')
   Post-parathyroidectomy for hyperparathyroidism
   Post-thyroidectomy
   Osteoblastic secondaries (lung, prostate, breast)
Acute pancreatitis
Renal failure
Hyperphosphataemia
   renal failure
   phosphate therapy
   tumour lysis
Drug therapy
   Frusemide, calcitonin, mithramycin, diphosphonates

Notes on hypocalcaemia

♦ **Mild hypocalcaemia (1.80–2.00 mmol/L)**

Causes: Transient, hypoalbuminaemia, renal failure, acute pancreatitis

Transient: Combination of biological variation & unavoidable labatory error. Normalises on retesting.
Low albumin: [Ca] usually >1.80 mmol/L
Renal failure: Low [Ca] associated with high [PO_4] & [Creat] (usually >0.40 mmol/L). Hypocalcaemia may be severe (below).
Pancreatitis: Fall occurs within 36 h of pain onset. Rarely falls below 1.80 mmol/L.

♦ **Severe hypocalcaemia (1.40–1.80 mmol/L)**

Causes: EDTA contamination, hypoparathyroidism, magnesium deficiency, renal failure, vitamin D deficiency syndromes

EDTA: Usually very low [Ca], eg <1.00 mmol/L, high [K], eg >10 mmol/L, & low ALP, eg <20 U/L.
Hypoparathyroid: Characterised by a very low [Ca], a high [PO_4], normal ALP, & low PTH, eg <2.0 pmol/L.
Mg deficiency: Inhibits PTH secretion & peripheral action. Characteristically associated with hypokalaemia and resistant to therapy until the subject is Mg replete. Common in acute & chronic alcoholism.
Vit D deficiency: Uncommon; charcterised by low [PO4], elevated ALP, and elevated PTH.
Renal failure: If severe &/or vtiamin D metabolism affected; values may fall below 1.80 mmol/L.

♦ **Rare & unusual causes of hypocalcaemia**

Tumour lysis, Osteoblastic metastases; Rhabdomyolysis; Drugs: anticonvulsants, calcitonin, mithramycin, phosphate therapy.

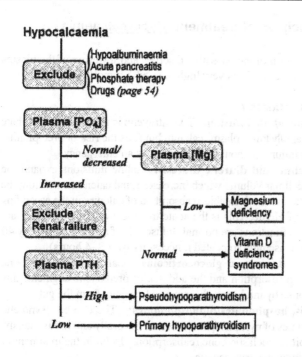

Hypocalcaemia

Exclude
- Hypoalbuminaemia
- Acute pancreatitis
- Phosphate therapy
- Drugs *(page 54)*

Plasma [PO$_4$]

Normal/decreased → Plasma [Mg]

Increased

Exclude Renal failure

Plasma PTH

Plasma [Mg]:
- *Low* → Magnesium deficiency
- *Normal* → Vitamin D deficiency syndromes

Plasma PTH:
- *High* → Pseudohypoparathyroidism
- *Low* → Primary hypoparathyroidism

Formular to correct for a low plasma albumin

Corrected [Ca] mmol/L =

Measured [Ca] mmol/L − 0.02(40−[Alb] g/L)

Evaluation of hypocalcaemia

Principles of treatment: <u>Hypercalcaemia</u>

Resolution of the causative disorder and lowering of the plasma calcium level if it is very high (e.g. >3.5 mmol/L).

Acute therapy
Phosphate infusion: The intravenous infusion of phosphate will rapidly lower plasma calcium but runs the risk of precipitating renal failure. It should only be used as an emergency.

Saline and diuretic diuresis: Saline infusions expand the extracellular volume which increases renal calcium excretion; the diuretic frusemide inhibits reabsorption of calcium in the ascending loop of Henle. This is the acute treatment of choice if renal and cardiac functions are normal. Infuse 2 L of saline followed by 40 mg of frusemide (repeated if necessary over 3–4 hours).

Calcitonin and glucocorticoids: Calcitonin inhibits bone calcium resorption and the addition of prednisone augments this response by inhibiting absorption of calcium from the gut.

Bisphosphonates/diphosphonates: These new synthetic analogues of pyrophosphate, active both orally and intravenously, inhibit osteoclastic bone reabsorption. Useful in the treatment of malignant hypercalcaemia.

Mithramycin: Inhibits bone resorption but may have serious side effects (thrombo-cytopenia, haemorrhage, renal impairment). Reserve for cases resistant to other types of therapy.

Chronic therapy
Maintain the plasma calcium at normal or near normal levels.by treating the causative disorder or using following medications.

.....................................*Cont'd next page*

(Treatment of hypercalcaemia continued)
Oral phosphate therapy: Phosphates bind calcium in the gut and prevent absorption. However, this method should not be used if there is renal insufficiency. **Steroid therapy:** Steroids probably act by decreasing calcium absorption. However, the administration of steroids as a long-term therapy is undesirable due to their known side effects (e.g. Cushing's syndrome). **Bisphosphonates:** These compounds are the most encouraging therapeutic agents presently available for the management of chronic hypercalcaemia.

Principles of treatment: <u>Hypocalcaemia</u>

Hypocalcaemia associated with tetany or carpopedal spasm should be treated with an ***intravenous infusion of calcium***. The usual procedure is to infuse 10-20 mL of 10% calcium gluconate over 2-3 minutes and repeat if necessary (calcium chloride is also available for infusion but is to be avoided because of the possibility of thrombophlebitis). *If the hypocalcaemic symptoms persist despite calcium infusion, the possibility of hypomagnesaemia should be considered.*

The *long-term treatment of hypocalcaemia* (e.g. that of hypoparathyroidism or severe vitamin D deficiency) should be managed by *vitamin D* therapy supplemented with oral *calcium*, e.g. vitamin D: dihydrotachysterol 15 mg daily, 1,25-dihydroxy-cholecalciferol (calcitriol): 2.5 µg daily; calcium: 2-4 g of elemental calcium daily. During treatment with these medications a careful watch should be kept on the plasma calcium levels because of the possibility of hypercalcaemia.

---

8 Phosphate

Hypophosphataemia *(see Figure page 61)*

> **Common causes of severe hypophosphataemia (<0.3 mmol/L)**
> ♦ Alcohol withdrawal syndrome
> ♦ Nutritional recovery syndrome
> ♦ Recovery after severe burns
> ♦ Aluminium hydroxide therapy
> ♦ Treatment of diabetic ketoacidosis
> ♦ Respiratory alkalosis
> ♦ Hyperalimentation

Decreased intake/GI loss
Starvation/inadequate IV nutrition; Malabsorption syndrome; Vomiting; Antacid therapy: *Phosphate binding with aluminium hydroxide*
Increased cell uptake
High carbohydrate intake; Nutritional recovery ; Insulin therapy; Alkalosis: *respiratory, metabolic;* Hungry-bone syndrome; Severe liver disease
Increased renal excretion
Diuretic therapy; Magnesium deficiency ; Renal phosphate leak: *Fanconi syndrome, vitamin D resistant rickets;* Hyperparathyroidism: *primary, secondary;* Malignant hypercalcaemia; Oncogenic hypophosphataemic osteomalacia
Multiple causes
Alcoholism, Diabetes mellitus, Burns, Hyperalimentation

Hypophosphataemia

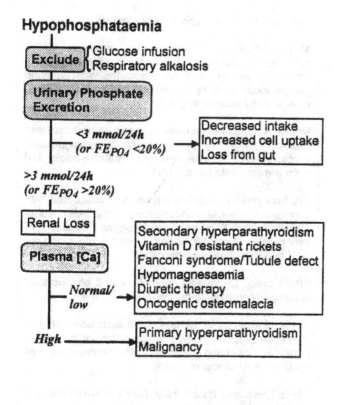

$$FE_{PO4}(\%) = \frac{Urine\ [PO_4]}{Plasma\ [PO_4]} \times \frac{Plasma\ [Creat]}{Urine\ [Creat]} \times 100$$

Evaluation of hypophosphataemia

Consequences of Hypophosphataemia

Mild phosphate depletion has minimal clinical consequences but severe depletion with plasma levels less than 0.20 mmol/L may be associated with profound complications involving the kidney, red and white blood cells, skeletal muscle, and bone.

Renal: A number of metabolic consequences have been described including hypercalciuria, hypermagnesuria, uricosuria, amino aciduria, decreased titratable acidity, and defective ammonia production.

Erythrocytes: Phosphate depletion is associated with diminished red cell concentrations of 2,3-diphosphoglycerate and thus decreased oxygen release from haemoglobin. Haemolytic anaemia, possibly due to red cell ATP depletion, has been described.

White cells: Decreased chemotaxis and phagocytosis accompany phosphate depletion.

Skeletal muscle: Weakness and muscle pain with mild rises in the plasma CK levels are common and respiratory paralysis has been described. Rhabdomyolysis has occurred in a number of cases.

CNS: There may be irritability. Coma, convulsions, and death have been observed.

Bone: Prolonged phosphate depletion will result in rickets and osteomalacia.

Hyperphosphataemia   *(see Figure page 65)*

Factitious
Delay in separation of red cells from plasma and/or haemolysis

Physiological
Infants and children

Increased intake
Oral/IV therapy, Vitamin D overdose

Release from cells
Tissue destruction: crush injury, rhabdomyolysis
Tumour lysis
Starvation
Acidaemia: respiratory, metabolic (lactic acidosis)
Insulin deficiency: diabetes mellitus
Bone release: primary or secondary malignancy
Malignant hyperthermia

Decreased renal excretion
Hypoparathyroidism: primary, pseudohypopara-
    thyroidism
Renal failure: acute, chronic
Growth hormone excess: acromegaly, giantism
Contraction of extracellular volume

Miscellaneous
Tumour calcinosis, Hypothyroidism, Intermittent primary
hyperphosphataemia, Post-menopausal hyperphosphataemia

Notes on hyperphosphataemia

Hyperphosphataemia is a common finding and may be a clue to the diagnosis of uncommon disorders such as hypoparathyroidism and vitamin D toxicity; however in clinical practice the majority of cases are due to:

- *Artifacts:* haemolysis, delayed separation of plasma from red cells

- *Renal failure*

- *'Hyperphosphataemia' of infancy and childhood:* the approximate normal ranges for this age group being:

Age	Reference range for plasma phosphate	
Neonates	1.2-2.8 mmol/L	(3.7-8.7 mg/dL)
<7 years	1.3-1.8 mmol/L	(4.0-5.6 mg/dL)
<15 years	0.7-1.2 mmol/L	(2.0-3.8 mg/dL)

Hyperphosphataemia

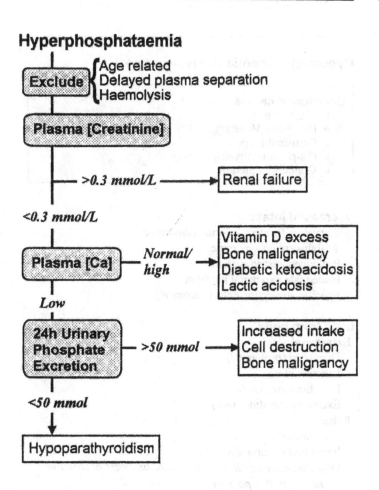

Evaluation of hyperphosphataemia

9 Magnesium

Hypomagnesaemia *(see Figure page 68)*

> **Commonest causes**
> ♦ Alcoholism
> ♦ Diarrhoea, Vomiting
> ♦ Diuretic therapy
> ♦ Cis-platinum therapy
> ♦ Gentamicin therapy

Decreased intake
Starvation (protein-calorie malnutrition)
Malabsorption syndrome
Prolonged gastric suction
Inadequate parenteral nutrition
Specific absorption defect (neonatal)

Loss from body
Extrarenal
Diarrhoea (prolonged)
Laxative abuse
Loss from gut fistula
Excessive lactation (rare)
Renal
Alcoholism
Interstitial nephropathy
Diuresis: *osmotic (diabetic ketoacidosis), post-obstructive nephropathy, post-ATN*
Drugs: *diuretics (especially loop), amphotericin B, gentamycin, cis-platinum, tobramycin, carbenicillin*
.... Cont'd over page

(Renal Loss Cont'd)
  Hypercalcaemia
  Renal tubular acidosis
  Bartter's syndrome, Gitelman's syndrome
  Endocrine: *primary hyperaldosteronism, hypopara-*
    thyroidism, hyperthyroidism, SIADH
  Post-renal transplant
  Primary renal magnesium loss
  Potassium depletion
  Phosphate depletion

Miscellaneous
  Acute pancreatitis (sequestration)
  Multiple transfusions (citrate precipitation)
  Insulin administration (redistribution)
  Hungry bone syndrome: *post-parathyroidectomy,*
    post-thyroidectomy

Notes on hypomagnesaemia/magnesium deficiency

Prevalence: 4%–5% of hospital population

Commonest presentation is transient hypomagnesaemia, ie [Mg] 0.50-0.70 mmol/L which normalises without specific therapy (often stress-related)

Biochemical complications
  • Hypokalaemia/potassium depletion
  • Hypocalcaemia
Both resistant to specific therapy until the subject is made magnesium replete.

Hypomagnesaemia

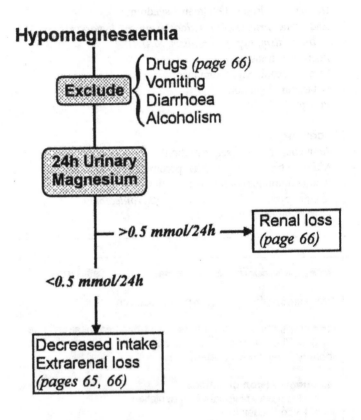

Evaluation of hypomagnesaemia

Principles of treatment: Magnesium Disorders

Hypomagnesaemia

In the acute situation magnesium can be given intravenously (25 mmol of magnesium sulphate in one litre of saline over three hours, repeated if necessary), or orally (up to 10 mmol of magnesium four times daily). Treatment should be continued for at least four days because (a) half of the administrated magnesium is lost in the urine, and (b) it takes some three to four days for a given dose of magnesium to distribute itself throughout the body. Plasma levels should be closely monitored and therapy ceased if the level rises above 2.0 mmol/L.

Hypermagnesaemia

Treatment of hypermagnesaemia involves decreasing the magnesium intake and, if necessary, antagonizing the toxic effects by calcium gluconate infusions. In severe cases dialysis may be required.

Hypermagnesaemia

Commonest causes
♦ Renal failure

NB Excepting IV magnesium infusions and severe renal failure, hypermagnesaemia usually results from increased intake *PLUS* decreased renal excretion.

Increased intake*

Oral: antacids, laxatives
IV magnesium therapy *e.g. treatment of eclampsia*
Dialysis: *fluid containing large concentrations of magnesium*

Cell release

Diabetic ketoacidosis
Severe anoxia *e.g. birth asphyxia*
Cell necrosis/catabolism

Decreased excretion

Renal failure: *acute, chronic.*
Familial hypocalciuric hypercalcaemia
Mineralocorticoid deficiency
Hypothyroidism

* usually only when associated with decreased renal excretion

10 Uric acid

Hyperuricaemia *(see Figure page 73)*

> **Commonest causes**
> ◆ Gout
> ◆ Potentially correctable conditions:
>   Ethanol consumption
>   Obesity
>   Hypertriglyceridaemia
>   Hypertension
>   Diuretic therapy
>   Drugs: *salicylates, nicotinic acid, pyrazinamide,*
>   *cyclosporin, ethambutol*
>   Starvation
>   Low urine volume/dehydration

Primary
Excess production (secretors, ~20%)
Idiopathic
Defects of: HGPRT, 5-phosphoribose 1-pyrophosphatesynthetase, glucose 6-phosphatase
Reduced excretion
Idiopathic

Secondary
Overproduction
Haematological: myeloproliferative disorders, chronic haemolytic anaemia, leukaemia, lymphomas, infectious mononucleosis, myeloma
Malignancy: rapidly growing, therapy (chemotherapy/ irradiation)
Increased cell turnover: psoriasis, starvation
Increased ATP turnover: alcohol, exercise

.... *Cont'd over page*

(Overproduction continued)
Reduced excretion
Renal failure
Lead nephropathy
Dehydration/low urine output
Diuretic therapy: thiazides, ethacrynic acid
Ketoacidosis: starvation, diabetes mellitus, ethanol
Lactic acidosis: ethanol, toxaemia of pregnancy
Drugs: salicylate (low dose), ethambutol, pyrazinamide, nicotinic
    acid, cyclosporin
Hyperparathyroidism
Myxoedema

HGPRT, hypoxanthine-guanine phosphoribosyl-transferase

Notes on gout

Prevalence of about 3 per 1000 of the general population of which 90% to 95% are men.

Characterised by one or more of the following:

- acute or chronic arthritis
- urate deposits (tophi) in subcutaneous tissues,
- joints, tendons
- renal calculi of uric acid
- urate nephropathy

Definitive diagnosis requires demonstration of uric acid crystals in tissues, eg in leucocytes from synovial fluid. **Note** During an acute gout attack the serum urate may not be elevated.

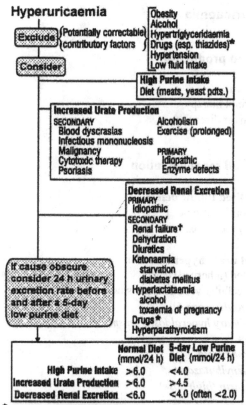

Hyperuricaemia

Exclude / Consider — Potentially correctable contributory factors

Obesity
Alcohol
Hypertriglyceridaemia
Drugs (esp. thiazides)*
Hypertension
Low fluid intake

High Purine Intake
Diet (meats, yeast pdts.)

Increased Urate Production

SECONDARY
Blood dyscrasias
Infectious mononucleosis
Malignancy
Cytotoxic therapy
Psoriasis

Alcoholism
Exercise (prolonged)

PRIMARY
Idiopathic
Enzyme defects

Decreased Renal Excretion

PRIMARY
   Idiopathic
SECONDARY
   Renal failure†
   Dehydration
   Diuretics
   Ketonaemia
      starvation
      diabetes mellitus
   Hyperlactataemia
      alcohol
      toxaemia of pregnancy
   Drugs*
   Hyperparathyroidism

If cause obscure consider 24 h urinary excretion rate before and after a 5-day low purine diet

	Normal Diet (mmol/24 h)	5-day Low Purine Diet (mmol/24 h)
High Purine Intake	>6.0	<4.0
Increased Urate Production	>6.0	>4.5
Decreased Renal Excretion	<6.0	<4.0 (often <2.0)

* Drugs: Diuretics, Salicylates (low dose), Nicotinic acid, Pyrazinamide, Ethambutol, Cyclosporin.

† Renal failure: If cause, then serum [creatinine] will be >0.40 mmol/L, serum [urate] <0.65 mmol/L & urine urate:creatinine ratio <0.7. If hyperuricaemia causing the renal failure then serum urate >0.7 mmol/L & urine urate:creat ratio >0.7.

Evaluation of hyperuricaemia

Hypouricaemia

Reduced production

Xanthinuria
Allopurinol therapy
Severe liver disease

Increased renal excretion

Generalised tubule defect
Fanconi syndrome
Heavy metal toxicity

Isolated urate hyperexcretion
Isolated (inherited) defect
Extracellular volume expansion
SIADH (page 6)
Primary hyperaldosteronism
Drugs
probenecid
phenylbutazone
aspirin (high dose)

Analytical interference

High plasma Vitamin C levels

11 Glucose

Hyperglycaemia *(see Figure page 76)*

> **Commonest causes**
> ♦ Postprandial
> ♦ Diabetes mellitus
> ♦ Stress
>
> **NB** Stress-realted hyperglycemia rarely exceeds 10 mmol/L

Postprandial

Carbohydrate intake: oral/intravenous
'Lag' storage: post-gastrectomy
            severe liver disease
            thyrotoxicosis

Fasting

Diabetes mellitus: insulin-dependent (IDDM),
   non-insulin-dependant (NIDDM)
Pancreatic disorders: pancreatectomy, haemochromatosis, chronic
   pancreatitis, carcinoma of pancreas
Endocrine causes: Cushing's syndrome, phaeochromocytoma,
   acromegaly, thyrotoxicosis
Stress reaction (temporary hyperglycaemia): trauma, shock,
   infection, cerebrovascular accident, myocardial infarction,
   burns
Drugs (temporary hyperglycaemia): salicylates, steroids,
   thiazides, oral contraceptives/oestrogens

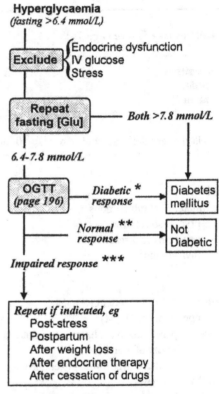

Hyperglycaemia
(fasting >6.4 mmol/L)

Exclude {Endocrine dysfunction / IV glucose / Stress}

Repeat fasting [Glu] —— *Both >7.8 mmol/L*

6.4–7.8 mmol/L

OGTT *(page 196)* —— *Diabetic* * *response* → Diabetes mellitus

Normal ** *response* → Not Diabetic

Impaired response ***

Repeat if indicated, eg
Post-stress
Postpartum
After weight loss
After endocrine therapy
After cessation of drugs

OGTT Oral glucose tolerance test
[Glu] plasma glucose concentration
* 2h [Glu] >11.1 mmol/L
** 2h [Glu] <7.8 mmol/L
*** 2h [Glu] 7.8–11.1 mmol/L

Evaluation of hyperglycaemia (Adult)

Monitoring therapy of Diabetes Mellitus

In addition to clinical observation and regular blood glucose estimations diabetic patients can benefit from regular estimations of blood **glycosylated haemoglobins** and **urinary microalbumin** excretion.

Glycosylated haemoglobins and proteins

Haemoglobin A_{1c} is formed by the non-enzymatic attachment of glucose to haemoglobin A. It is formed continuously throughout the 120-day life-span of the red cell and provides an index of the 'average' plasma glucose concentration over the preceding two to three months. It is useful for assessing diabetic control. The values reflecting control in diabetics will vary significantly from laboratory to laboratory, eg.

Near normal glycaemia	6.0–7.0%
Excellent control	7.0–8.0%
Good control	8.0–9.0%
Fair control	9.0–10.0%
Poor control	>10%

A number of plasma proteins including albumin also become glycosylated during hyperglycaemia. These are measured in the laboratory as plasma fructosamine and reflect the average blood glucose concentration over the preceding one to three weeks. However due to its variability plasma fructosamine has not found wide acceptance in the monitoring of diabetics.

.... *Cont'd next page*

Urinary microalbumin

Microalbumin (small amounts not small molecules) is defined as small elevations of urinary albumin excretion not detected by conventional means (eg albustix).. Increased levels imply early kidney disease. Useful screening procedure for the detection of early renal complications of diabetes mellitus and hypertension.

The accepted method of estimation is the albumin excretion rate (AER, μg/min). This requires an accurately timed urine sample; best performed overnight(exercise can increase excretion rate). Length of collection in not important but the exact timing is paramount. An albumin:creatinine ratio (mg/L:mmol/L) on an early morning spot urine is an acceptable screening method; equivocal or increased ratios must be followed by a timed sample for AER estimation. The appropriate *reference ranges* are:

Albumin excretion rate (AER):   <15 μg/min
Albumin:creatinine ratio: <3.5
Albumin concentration: <20 μg/mL

An AER in excess of 30 μg/min is considered to indicate significant renal disease (but this not only cause of elevation):

Persistent: *Renal disease* (Diabetic, Hypertensive)
          CCF (anoxia, increased filtration pressure)
          Chronic lung disease (? Renal anoxia)
          Malignancy (? cause)
Transient: (5–15 x normal values)
          Post exercise (up to 30 μg/mL)
          Post surgery*, Trauma*, Septicaemia*,
          Acute pancreatitis*, Myocardial infarction*

* Occurs within 60 min and lasts 1-48 h. (Parallels C-reactive protein but appears earlier)

Hypoglycaemia - adults *(see Figure page 80)*

Commonest causes
- Exogenous insulin
- Oral hypoglycaemics
- Insulinoma

In one survey of 204 episodes of hypoglycaemia 200 were due to insulin therapy, three to oral hypoglycaemics, and one to insulinoma.

Exogenous causes
Insulin therapy/abuse
Oral hypoglycaemic therapy/abuse
Ethanol
Drugs: *salicylates, β-adrenergic blockers*

Endogenous causes - Reactive
Idiopathic (functional)
Early diabetes mellitus (adult onset)
Alimentary (gastric surgery)

Endogenous causes - Fasting
Insulinoma
Non-pancreatic tumours *(fibroma, fibrosarcoma,*
    hepatoma, adrenal carcinoma)
Hypopituitarism
Liver failure
Renal failure
Sepsis
Autoimmune hypoglycaemia *(insulin antibodies,*
    insulin receptor antibodies)

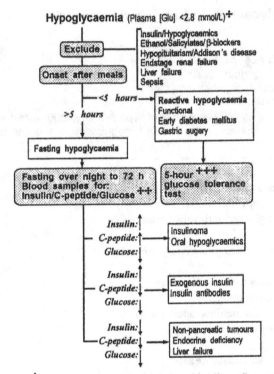

Hypoglycaemia (Plasma [Glu] <2.8 mmol/L)[+]

Exclude:
- Insulin/Hypoglycaemics
- Ethanol/Salicylates/ β-blockers
- Hypopituitarism/Addison's disease
- Endstage renal failure
- Liver failure
- Sepsis

Onset after meals

<*5 hours* →

Reactive hypoglycaemia
Functional
Early diabetes mellitus
Gastric sugery

>*5 hours*

Fasting hypoglycaemia

Fasting over night to 72 h
Blood samples for:
Insulin/C-peptide/Glucose [++]

5-hour [+++]
glucose tolerance
test

Insulin: ↑
C-peptide: ↑ → Insulinoma / Oral hypoglycaemics
Glucose: ↓

Insulin: ↑
C-peptide: ↓ → Exogenous insulin / Insulin antibodies
Glucose: ↓

Insulin: ↓
C-peptide: ↓ → Non-pancreatic tumours / Endocrine deficiency / Liver failure
Glucose: ↓

[+] If performed on serum or plasma, check result by taking another sample into a fluoride container as *in vitro* glycolysis can result in a low glucose

[++] Measure blood glucose after an overnight fast on several occasions; if glucose not <2.8 mmol/L continue fast for up to 72 h taking blood for glucose, Insulin and C-peptide at 4 h intervals or if symptoms occur.

[+++] GTT to exclude diabetes/glucose intolerance. If hypoglycaemia occurs repeat test using a mixed meal instead of glucose as 10-20% of normal subjects will develop hypoglycaemia after a glucose load.

Evaluation of adult hypoglycaemia

Hypoglycaemia - infants & children *(Figure page 83)*

> **Commonest causes**
> *Newborn*: Intrauterine growth retardation
> Diabetic mother
> Birth asphyxia/infectiom
> *Children*: Exogenous insulin/oral hypoglycaemics
> Metabolic defects

Neonatal
Transient

↓ Insulin: Small for dates baby
Sepsis/asphyxia/cerebral haemorrhage

↑ Insulin: Diabetic mother
Erythroblastosis fetalis
Beckwith-Widemann syndrome

Persistent

↓ insulin: Enzyme defects *(see page 82)*
Hormone deficiencies: *growth hormone, thyroxine,
glucagon*

↑ Insulin: Nesidoblastosis
Islet cell adenoma
Leucine sensitivity
Beckwith-Widemann syndrome

Infancy (first year of life)
As for neonatal persistent

.... *Cont'd over page*

(Hypoglycaemia continued)
Childhood
↓ Insulin: Ketotic hypoglycaemia
              Enzyme defects *(see below)*
              Hormone deficiencies *(see above)*
              Reye's syndrome
              Salicylate overdose
              Ethanol intoxication
              Non-pancreatic tumours

↑ Insulin: Islet cell adenoma/hyperplasia
              Exogenous insulin
              Oral hypoglycaemics

Enzyme defects associated with hypoglycaemia

Carbohydrate
Glycogenesis: glycogen synthetase, glucose 6- phosphatase,
    debrancher enzyme, glycogen phosphorylase
Gluconeogenesis: pyruvate carboxylase, phosphoenolpyruvate
    carboxykinase, fructose bisphosphatase, glucose 6-phosphatase
Others: fructose 1,6-bisphosphate aldolase (fructose intolerance),
    UDP-glucose galactose 1-phosphate uridyl transferase
    (galactosaemia)
Amino acids
branched chain ketoacid dehydrogenase (maple syrup disease)
Fatty acids
carnitine palmityltransferase, acetyl-CoA dehydrogenase (medium,
short, and long chain), HMG-CoA lyase, carnitine deficiency
Organic acidurias
propionic aciduria, methylmalonic aciduria

Hypoglycaemia

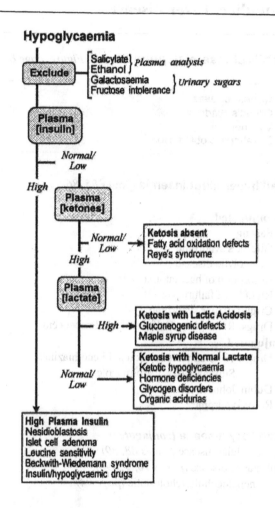

Evaluation of hypoglycaemia in children

12 Jaundice, Liver disease

Hyperbilirubinaemia/Jaundice *(see Figure page 85)*

Commonest causes
- Gilbert's syndrome
- Viral hepatitis
- Extrahepatic obstruction

Isolated hyperbilirubinaemia *(pages 85, 86)*

Unconjugated
Fasting
Gilbert's syndrome
Haemolytic disease
Resorption of haematoma
Right heart failure
Crigler-Najjar syndrome
Drugs: Rifampicin, Sulfonamides, Probenecid

Conjugated
Drugs: 17-α-alkylated steroids, Phenothiazines,
Sulfonamides, Carbimazole
Dubin-Johnson syndrome
Rotor syndrome

Hepatobiliary disease *(conjugated)*
Hepatocellular disease *(pages 88, 89)*
Cholestastic disease *(pages 90, 92, 93)*
Mixed hepatocellular/cholestatic *(page 94)*

Jaundice

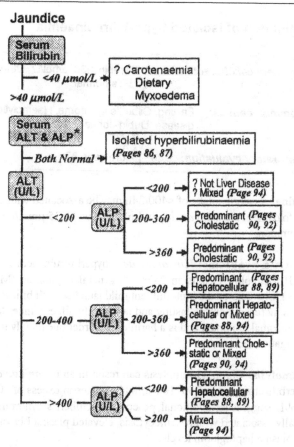

*The values quoted are "rule-of-thumb" and suggestions only.

Evaluation of the jaundiced patient.
(ALT alanine aminotransferase, ALP alkaline phosphatase)

Evaluation of isolated hyperbilirubinaemia.

Biochemical characteristics:	Bilirubin >30 µmol/L; Other LFTs normal
Common causes:	Fasting, Gilbert's syndrome, Haemolytic disease, Dubin-Johnson syndrome
Laboratory evaluation:	see Figure page 87.

Fasting: A calorie intake of <400/24h may be assocaited with a 2 to 3-fold rise in *unconjugated* bilirubin but values >35 µmol/L are uncommon.

Gilbert's syndrome: *Unconjugated* hyperbilirubinaemia of 25–100 µmol/L. Occurs in 2–7% of general population (M:F 2–7:1). Characterised by intermittent mild jaundice with bilirubin values increasing during fasting and nonspecific illness. Inherited as autosomal dominant and is a harmless disorder due mainly to a conjugation defect.

Haemolysis: Chronic haemolysis can result in an *unconjugated* hyperbilirubinaemia of 50–100 µmol/L; values in excess of 100 µmol/L suggest an additional process, eg Gilbert's syndrome. Usually associated with reticulocytosis, elevated plasma LD, and low plasma haptoglobin levels.

Dubin–Johnson syndrome: A rare autosomal recessive disorder associated with fluctuating *conjugated* hyperbilirubinaemia (up to 100 µmol/L) and a characteristic deep green pigmentation of the liver. Due to inability to excrete conjugated bilirubin; harmless.

Isolated Hyperbilirubinaemia

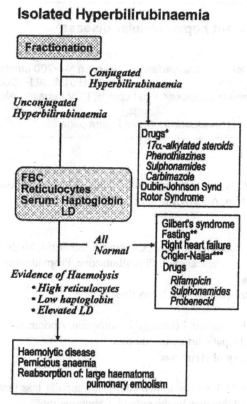

Fractionation

Conjugated Hyperbilirubinaemia

Unconjugated Hyperbilirubinaemia

Drugs*
17α-alkylated steroids
Phenothiazines
Sulphonamides
Carbimazole
Dubin-Johnson Synd
Rotor Syndrome

**FBC
Reticulocytes
Serum: Haptoglobin
LD**

All Normal →

Gilbert's syndrome
Fasting**
Right heart failure
Crigler-Najjar***
Drugs
  Rifampicin
  Sulphonamides
  Probenecid

Evidence of Haemolysis
  • *High reticulocytes*
  • *Low haptoglobin*
  • *Elevated LD*

Haemolytic disease
Pernicious anaemia
Reabsorption of: large haematoma
                 pulmonary embolism

* Usually associated with increased ALT and ALP
** Bilirubin usually <40 μmol/L & fasting >24 hours
*** Uncommon disorder usually diagnosed at birth

FBC full blood count (examination), LD lactate dehydrogenase

Evaluation of isolated hyperbilirubinaemia

Predominant hepatocellular disease

> *Biochemical characteristics:* Bilirubin N→>200 μmol/L
> ALT >150 U/L, ALP <200 U/L.
> *Commonest causes:* Viral hepatitis, EBV hepatitis, Alcohol,
> Drugs,
> *Laboratory evaluation:* see Figure page 89.

Infection
Hepatitis A, B, C[1], EBV infection, Cytomegalovirus, Coxsackie
virus infection, Adenovirus infection
Alcohol[2]
Drugs
Amxocillin, Chlortetracycline, Cytotoxics, Isoniazid, Methyldopa,
Methotrexate, Paracetamol, Phenylbutazone, Propylthiouracil
Chemicals
Carbon tetrachloride, Trichloroethylene
Anoxia
Acute cardiac failure, Prolonged hypotension, Abdominal
aneurysm, Hepatic artery thrombosis
Acute biliary obstruction[3]

[1] Plasma ALT values in hepatitis C are usually less than 200
IU/L and this may be the only LFT abnormality
[2] In alcoholic liver disease the transaminases (ALT, AST) are
usually less than 300 IU/L and often the AST value is greater
the ALT value
[3] Transient rise in transaminases (up to 1000 U/L) early in
disease prior to rise in ALP.

Predominant Hepatocellular Pathology

$$\left.\begin{array}{l} \text{1. ALT or AST >150 U/L} \\ \text{2. ALP <200 U/L} \end{array}\right\} \pm \text{Jaundice}$$

Infection
Hepatitis A, B, C
EBV infection
Cytomegalovirus → Viral Studies
Coxsakie infection
Adenovirus infection

Acute biliary* → Clinical assessment
obstruction Radiology

Alcohol** → •AST & ALT <400 U/L
•AST>ALT
Drugs † •GGT: ↑**
Amoxycillin
Chlortetracycline
Cytotoxics
Isoniazid → Clinical
Methyldopa assessment
Methotrexate
Paracetamol
Phenylbutazone
Propylthiouracil

Chemicals † → Clinical
Carbontetrachloride assessment
Trichlorethylene

Anoxia
Acute cardiac failure
Prolonged hypotension → Clinical
Abdominal aneurysm assessment
Hepatic artery thrombosis

* Transient rise in ALT & AST early in the disease before
  rise in ALP becomes evident (values may be >1000 U/L).
** In alcoholic hepatitis ALT is usually less than 300 U/L and
   often less than 200 U/L; AST often greater than ALT
† Common agents only; list not comprehensive.

Evaluation of hepatocellular disease.

(ALT alanine aminotransferase, ALP alkaline phosphatase, GGT gamma-glutamyltransferase)

Cholestatic (obstructive) hepatobiliary disease.

> **Biochemical characteristics:** Bilirubin 40→200 µmol/L.
> ALT <400 U/L, ALP >350 U/L.
> **Commonest causes:** Cholelithiasis, Malignancy, Drugs,
> Cirrhosis
> **Laboratory evaluation:** see Figure page 92.

Canicular cholestasis*

Drugs: Oestrogens/oral contraceptives;
Androgens: *Methyl-testosterone, Danazol*
Phenothiazines, Tricyclics, Benzodiazepines
Erythromycin
Miscellaneous: Gold, Captopril, Carbimazole,
Azathioprine, Sulphonylureas, Phenylbutazone
Hepatitis: Viral, Alcoholic
Bacterial Infections: Gram negative septicaemia
Pregnancy
Post-operative cholestasis
Benign recurrent cholestasis

Interlobular bile duct cholestasis*

Primary biliary cirrhosis
Sclerosing cholangitis
Postnecrotic cirrhosis
Total parenteral nutrition

* Usually associated with jaundice (*Figure page 92*)

.... *Cont'd next page*

(Cholestatic jaundice continued)
Intrahepatic bile duct cholestasis/multifocal lesions**
Carcinoma: Secondary, Primary
Granulomas: Sarcoid, Tuberculosis
Abscess/Cyst
Lymphoma/Hodgkin's disease
Sclerosing cholangitis
Intraduct papillomatosis
Intraduct lithiasis
Extrahepatic bile duct cholestasis*
Choledocolithiasis
Biliary stricture
Pancreatitis
Periampullary carcinoma

** Jaundice usually absent (localised cholestasis, *Figure page 93*)
   unless severe or wide spread.
* Usually associated with jaundice (*Figure page 92*).

Mild localised cholestasis of uncertain origin

Biochemical features: ALT: Normal, ALP: 140-200 U/L
                        GGT: 100-300 U/L
Consider:
Fatty infiltration (steatosis)
Portal triaditis: Nonspecific mild inflammation of portal tracts
Acute extrahepatic infections: Transient elevation of
                               liver-related ALP (? Acute
                               phase reaction)
Two disorders: eg, bone-related ALP (Paget's disease,
                malignancy) PLUS elevated GGT due to
                enzyme induction (alcohol, drugs, page
                103)

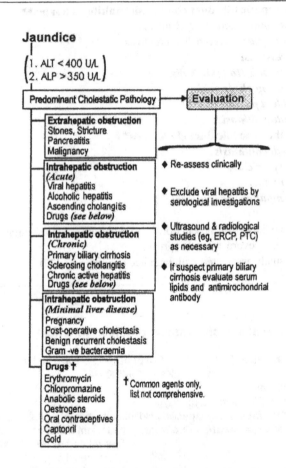

Jaundice

$$\begin{pmatrix} 1.\ ALT < 400\ U/L \\ 2.\ ALP > 350\ U/L \end{pmatrix}$$

Predominant Cholestatic Pathology → **Evaluation**

Extrahepatic obstruction
Stones, Stricture
Pancreatitis
Malignancy

Intrahepatic obstruction
(Acute)
Viral hepatitis
Alcoholic hepatitis
Ascending cholangitis
Drugs *(see below)*

Intrahepatic obstruction
(Chronic)
Primary biliary cirrhosis
Sclerosing cholangitis
Chronic active hepatitis
Drugs *(see below)*

Intrahepatic obstruction
(Minimal liver disease)
Pregnancy
Post-operative cholestasis
Benign recurrent cholestasis
Gram -ve bacteraemia

Drugs †
Erythromycin
Chlorpromazine
Anabolic steroids
Oestrogens
Oral contraceptives
Captopril
Gold

† Common agents only,
list not comprehensive.

◆ Re-assess clinically

◆ Exclude viral hepatitis by
serological investigations

◆ Ultrasound & radiological
studies (eg, ERCP, PTC)
as necessary

◆ If suspect primary biliary
cirrhosis evaluate serum
lipids and antimirochondrial
antibody

Evaluation of Cholestatic jaundice.

(ALT alanine aminotransferase, ALP alkaline phosphatase. ERCP
endoscopic retrograde cholangiopancreatography, PTC percutaneous
transhepatic cholangiography.)

Localised Cholestasis

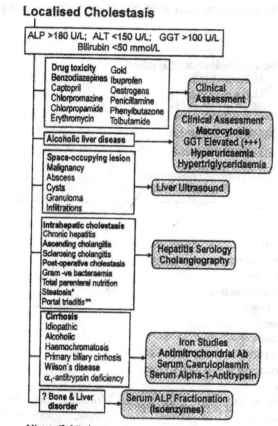

Evaluation of localised cholestasis

(ALP alkaline phosphatase, ALT alanine aminotransferase, GGT gamma-glutamyltransferase)

Mixed hepatocellular and cholestatic pathology

Biochemical characteristics
ALT: >150 U/L
ALP: >200 U/L
Bilirubin: Variable

Commonest Causes
♦ Malignancy
♦ Drugs
♦ Prolonged obstruction

Hepatitis
Acute (cholestatic variety)
Alcoholic
Biliary obstruction
Prolonged
Cirrhosis
Decompensated
Malignancy
Secondary
Drugs
p-Amino salicylic acid, Chlorambucil, Halothane, Ibuprofen, α-Methyldopa, Nitrofurantoin, Penicillamine, Pheylbutazone, Phenytoin, Sulfonamides, Valproate

Other possibility
Bone disease (high ALP) associated with hepatocellular disease (high ALT). An ALP fractionation should resolve the issue.

Neonatal jaundice

Presenting within first 10 days
Unconjugated hyperbilirubinaemia
Physiological jaundice
Breast milk jaundice
Haemolytic disease: *Blood group incompatibility (Rhesus, ABO, Kell), Glucose 6-phodphate dehydrogenase deficiency, Hereditary spherocytosis*
Hypothyroidism
Gilbert's disease
Crigler-Najjar syndrome
Conjugated hyperbilirubinaemia
Dubin-Johnson syndrome
Rotor syndrome
Biliary atresia
Alagille syndrome
Cystic fibrosis
Neonatal hepatitis: *Rubella, Toxoplasma, Cytomegalovirus, Herpes, Hepatitis A & B, Coxsakie, Syphilis*
Inborn errors of metabolism: *Galactosaemia, Fructose intolerance, Tyrosinaemia, α_1-antitrypsin deficiency*
Lipidoses: *Niemann-Pick disease, Gaucher's disease*

Presenting after or lasting more than 10 days
Breast milk jaundice, Infection, Biliary atresia, Alagille syndrome, α_1-antitrypsin deficiency, Hypothyroidism, Inborn errors of metabolism, Cystic fibrosis, Crigler-Najjar syndrome, Total parenteral nutrition

13 Enzymes

Hyperphosphatasaemia *(see Figure page 98)*

> **Commonest causes**
> ♦ Hepatobiliary disease
> ♦ Renal osteodystrophy
> ♦ Paget's disease

Physiological
Age: *neonates, children, young adults*
Pregnancy: *third trimester*

Liver disease
Hepatocellular *(page 88)*
Cholestasis *(page 90, 93)*
Space-occupying lesions: tumour, cyst, granuloma, abscess

Bone disease
Paget's disease
Malignancy: *primary, secondary*
Hyperparathyroidism: *primary, secondary*
Chronic renal failure: *renal osteodystrophy*
Rickets/osteomalacia
Healing fractures

Malignancy
Bone: *primary, secondary*
Liver: *primary, secondary*
Ectopic production: *Regan isoenzyme*

.... *Cont'd over page*

(Hyperphosphatasaemia continued)
Miscellaneous
    Transient hyperphosphatasaemia of infancy
    Familial benign hyperphosphatasaemia
    Hyperthyroidism
    Congestive cardiac failure
    IV therapy: *albumin prepared from placentas,*
    Parenteral nutrition
    Extrahepatic infections (?acute phase reaction)

Reference ranges

Age
The normal plasma ALP levels vary with age. Typical reference ranges are:

Birth	30-100 U/L
1 month	70-250 U/L
1-3 years	70-220 U/L
3-10 years	75-340 U/L
10-16 years	40-340 U/L
Adults	30-120 U/L

Regardless of the above values, rapidly growing children may present with plasma ALP values of the order of 500-1000 U/L.

Pregnancy

    150-300 U/L (during third trimester)

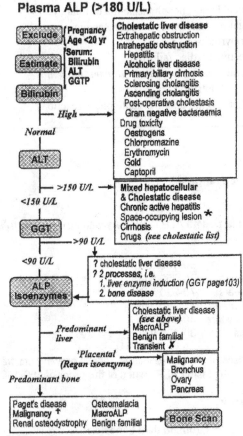

Plasma ALP (>180 U/L)

Exclude { Pregnancy / Age <20 yr

Estimate { Serum: / Bilirubin / ALT / GGTP

Bilirubin

— *High* →

Cholestatic liver disease
Extrahepatic obstruction
Intrahepatic obstruction
  Hepatitis
  Alcoholic liver disease
  Primary biliary cirrhosis
  Sclerosing cholangitis
  Ascending cholangitis
  Post-operative cholestasis
  Gram negative bacteraemia
Drug toxicity
  Oestrogens
  Chlorpromazine
  Erythromycin
  Gold
  Captopril

Normal

ALT

— *>150 U/L* →

Mixed hepatocellular & Cholestatic disease
Chronic active hepatitis
Space-occupying lesion *
Cirrhosis
Drugs *(see cholestatic list)*

<150 U/L

GGT

— *>90 U/L* →

? cholestatic liver disease
? 2 processes, i.e.
  1. liver enzyme induction (GGT page103)
  2. bone disease

<90 U/L

ALP Isoenzymes

Predominant liver →

Cholestatic liver disease
  (see above)
MacroALP
Benign familial
Transient ✗

'Placental (Regan isoenzyme) →

Malignancy
Bronchus
Ovary
Pancreas

Predominant bone

Paget's disease	Osteomalacia
Malignancy †	MacroALP
Renal osteodystrophy	Benign familial

Bone Scan

* Malignancy (primary, secondary), abscess, cyst
✗ Part of 'acute phase' reaction in extrahepatic infections
† Prostate, breast, kidney, myeloma, lymphoma, etc.

Evaluation of hyperphosphatasaemia

Hyperamylasaemia

Commonest causes
- Acute pancreatitis
- Gut obstruction/perforations
- Renal failure
- Macroamylaseamia

Pancreatic disorders
Acute pancreatitis: *alcohol-related, biliary tract disease,*
Trauma,
Hyperlipidaemia (types I, IV, V),
Carcinoma
Drugs: *thiazides, frusemide, azathioprin, glucocorticoids*

Non-pancreatic abdominal disease
Perforated peptic ulcer
Intestinal obstruction
Ischaemia of small bowel
Ruptured ectopic pregnancy
Salpingitis

Miscellaneous
Salivary glands: *mumps, duct obstruction*
Tumours: *carcinoma of bronchus, ovary, colon*
Renal failure
Diabetic ketoacidosis
Macroamylasaemia
Drugs: *opiates*

Persistent hyperamylasaemia

Pancreas
Persistent acute pancreatitis
Complications of pancreatitis: *pseudocyst, ascites, abscess*
Carcinoma

Non-pancreatic
Salivary glands: *tumours, infections (mumps), calculi*
Renal insufficiency
Macroamylasaemia
Tumours: *carcinoma of bronchus, colon, ovary*
Salpingitis

Notes on acute pancreatitis
In uncomplicated acute pancreatitis the serum amylase begins to rise within 1–2 hour of pain onset, reaches values in excess of three-times the upper limit of normal, and to normal level in 12–24 hours (half-life of about 12 hours).

Two important points:
1. Acute pancreatitis may be associated with a normal serum amylase:
   a. Blood specimen taken before or after rise
   b. Acute haemorrhagic pancreatitis — release to blood impeded by surrounding clot
2. Non-pancreatic abdominal diseases such as gut obstruction, gut perforations, ruptured ectopic pregnancy, can result is serum values similat to that of acute pancreatitis.

Transaminases - High serum levels

Aspartate aminotransferase (AST)
Myocardial disease
  Myocardial infarction, Myocarditis
Liver disease
  Hepatocellular disorders *(page 88)*
Skeletal muscle disease
  Muscular dystrophy, Trauma,
  Dermatomyositis, Myoglobinuria
Miscellaneous
  Haemolysis, Pernicious anaemia, Renal infarction,
  Acute pancreatitis, Malignancy: necrosis

Alanine aminotransferase
Can be considered as a specific liver enzyme *(pages 88, 89)*

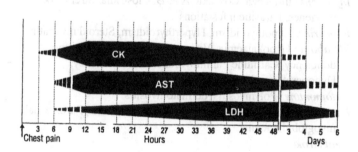

CK creatine kinase, AST aspartate aminotransferase, LDH lactate
dehydrogenase

Myocardial infarct: Enzyme time relationships

Creatine kinase (CK) - Elevated serun levels

Useful Laboratory Investigations
- Serum LD & AST
- CK-isoenzymes
- Urinary myoglobin
- Thyroid function tests
- Autoimmune serology

Cardiac muscle
Infarction, Myopathy, Myocarditis
Skeletal muscle
Injury/trauma: Crush, Surgery, IM injections, Ischaemia
Alcohol: Acute, Chronic
Drugs: Amphotericin B, Azathioprine, Chloroquine, Clofibrate, Colchicine, Cyclosporin, Opoids, Simvastatin, Steroids, Vincristine, Verapamil
Infections: Influenza, Coxsakie A & B, Clostridia, Streptococcus pyogenes, Parasitic infestations
Endocrine: Hypothyroidism, Hyperthyroidism, Steroid myopathy.
Metabolic: Hypokalaemia, Vitamin D deficiency, Carnitine deficiency, Carnitine Palmitoyltransferase deficiency, Hypoparathyroidism
Autoimmune: Polymyositis, dermatomyositis
Exercise: Severe exertion, Marathon run, Convulsions, Paroxysmal myoglobulinaemia
Heat stroke
Malignant hyperpyrexia
Muscle dystrophy
Miscellaneous
Macro-CK, Malignancy, Cerebrovascular disease & head injury, Diabetic ketoacidosis.

Gamma-glutamyltransferase (GGT) - Elevated serum levels *(see Figure page 105)*

> **Commonest causes**
> ♦ Alcohol
> ♦ Drugs: Phenytoin sodium
> ♦ Hepatobiliary disease
> ♦ Idiopathic
>
> *NB There can be significant liver disease without an elevated serum GGT*

Hepato-biliary diseases
Hepatocellular destruction *(page 88)*, Cholestasis *(page 90)*

Hepatic enzyme induction
Alcohol
Drugs: *Barbiturates, Phenytoin, Simvastatin, Tricyclics, Benzodiazepines, Warfarin*

Miscellaneous (? minimal liver damage)
Myocardial infarction
Congestive cardiac failure
Diabetes mellitus
Acute pancreatitis
Obesity

Idiopathic
Some "normal" subjects have elevated values up to around 150 U/L for no obvious reason.

Notes on gammaglutamyl transferase

Reference Range
- <40 U/L
- Some "normal" subjects have values up to 120-150 U/L for no obvious reason

Elevated levels
- Hepato-biliary disease
- Alcohol
- Drugs
- Non-specific disease

Hepato-biliary disease
Usually elevated in all disorders but *can have significant disease without an elevated GGTP*

Alcohol
- Increased in 30-90% of chronic/heavy drinkers due to (a) enzyme induction or (b) liver disease
- Usually normal in acute alcohol intake
- Significant decrease will not occur until ~7 days abstinence (serum half-life of ~26 days)

Drugs
Enzyme induction may be associated with: *Phenytoin Barbiturates, Warfarin, Benzodiazepines, Tricyclics, Simvastatin*

Non-specific disease
High serum values may be associated with: *Obesity, Diabetes mellitus, Hypertriglyceridaemia*(some authorities suggest that this may represent early fatty changes in the liver).

Elevated serum GGT (>100 U/L)

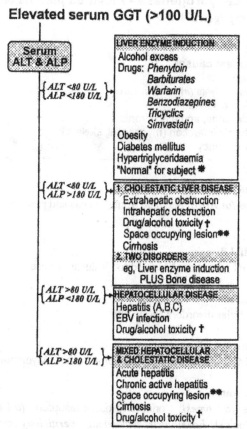

Serum ALT & ALP		
{ ALT <80 U/L ALP <180 U/L }	**LIVER ENZYME INDUCTION** Alcohol excess Drugs: *Phenytoin* *Barbiturates* *Warfarin* *Benzodiazepines* *Tricyclics* *Simvastatin* Obesity Diabetes mellitus Hypertriglyceridaemia "Normal" for subject *	

LIVER ENZYME INDUCTION
Alcohol excess
Drugs: *Phenytoin*
　　　Barbiturates
　　　Warfarin
　　　Benzodiazepines
　　　Tricyclics
　　　Simvastatin
Obesity
Diabetes mellitus
Hypertriglyceridaemia
"Normal" for subject *

{ ALT <80 U/L
ALP >180 U/L }

1. CHOLESTATIC LIVER DISEASE
　　Extrahepatic obstruction
　　Intrahepatic obstruction
　　Drug/alcohol toxicity †
　　Space occupying lesion **
　　Cirrhosis
2. TWO DISORDERS
　　eg, Liver enzyme induction
　　　　PLUS Bone disease

{ ALT >80 U/L
ALP <180 U/L }

HEPATOCELLULAR DISEASE
Hepatitis (A,B,C)
EBV infection
Drug/alcohol toxicity †

{ ALT >80 U/L
ALP >180 U/L }

**MIXED HEPATOCELLULAR
& CHOLESTATIC DISEASE**
Acute hepatitis
Chronic active hepatitis
Space occupying lesion **
Cirrhosis
Drug/alcohol toxicity †

* Some normal subjects have GGT values up to 150 U/L
** Space occupying lesions: malignancy, abscess, cyst etc
† In alcoholic liver disease the AST is often > ALT

Evaluation of an elevated GGT

Lactate dehydrogenase - Elevated plasma level
(see Figure page 107)

Commonest causes
- Factitious
- Haemolysis *(in vivo, in vitro)*
- Liver disease
- Infections, acute & chronic
- Muscle infarction (myocardial, skeletal)
- Malignancy

Factitious
Haemolysis *(in vitro)*; Seepage from red cells and platelets during clotting.

Myocardial disease
Myocardial infarction, Myocarditis, Valuvar disease

Liver disease
Hepatocellular disorders *(page 88)*

Skeletal muscle disease
Trauma, Muscular dystrophy, Dermatomyositis, Myoglobinuria

Miscellaneous
Infections: *(all types)*; Connective tissue disorders: *(all types)*; Haematological: *haemolysis, leukaemia, pernicious anaemia, myeloproliferative disorders*; Malignancy *(all types)*; Renal infarction; Pulmonary embolus; Hypothyroidism; Acute pancreatitis

---

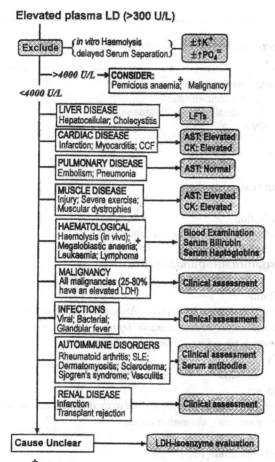

Elevated plasma LD (>300 U/L)

Exclude { *in vitro* Haemolysis / delayed Serum Separation } ±↑K⁺ / ±↑PO₄⁻

—>4000 U/L → CONSIDER: Pernicious anaemia;⁺ Malignancy

<4000 U/L

LIVER DISEASE
Hepatocellular; Cholecystitis → LFTs

CARDIAC DISEASE
Infarction; Myocarditis; CCF → AST: Elevated / CK: Elevated

PULMONARY DISEASE
Embolism; Pneumonia → AST: Normal

MUSCLE DISEASE
Injury; Severe exercise; Muscular dystrophies → AST: Elevated / CK: Elevated

HAEMATOLOGICAL
Haemolysis (in vivo); Megaloblastic anaemia;⁺ Leukaemia; Lymphoma → Blood Examination / Serum Bilirubin / Serum Haptoglobins

MALIGNANCY
All malignancies (25-80% have an elevated LDH) → Clinical assessment

INFECTIONS
Viral; Bacterial; Glandular fever → Clinical assessment

AUTOIMMUNE DISORDERS
Rheumatoid arthritis; SLE; Dermatomyositis; Scleroderma; Sjogren's syndrome; Vasculitis → Clinical assessment / Serum antibodies

RENAL DISEASE
Infarction
Transplant rejection → Clinical assessment

Cause Unclear —— LDH-Isoenzyme evaluation

⁺ Values in Pernicious Anaemia may exceed 9000 U/L.

Evaluation of an elevated LD

14 Serum proteins

Hyperproteinaemia *(see Figure page 110)*

> **Commonest causes**
> ♦ Haemoconcentration
> ♦ Polyclonal hyperglobulinaemia
> ♦ Myeloma

Haemoconcentration

Dehydration
Prolonged application of tourniquet

Hypergammaglobulinaemia

Polyclonal
Chronic liver disease: *cirrhosis, chronic active hepatitis*
Chronic infection: *bronchiectasis, leprosy, brucellosis,*
    tuberculosis, parasitic (malaria, Kala-azar)
Crohn's disease
Ulcerative colitis
Sarcoidosis
Autoimmune disorders: *rheumatoid arthritis, systemic lupus*
    erythrematosus, dermatomyositis

Monoclonal, malignant
Myelomatosis
Soft tissue plasmacytoma
Macroglobulinaemia

.... *Cont'd next page*

(Monoclonal, malignant Cont'd)
Heavy chain disease
Lymphoreticular malignancy: *lymphosarcoma, leukaemia, Hodgkin's disease*

Monoclonal, benign
Idiopathic *(monoclonal gammopathy of unknown significance)*
Secondary *to: diabetes mellitus, chronic infections, liver cirrhosis, connective tissue disorders*

Notes on hyperproteinaemia

1. The only cause of a high serum albumin concentration is haemoconcentration:

   ♦ Dehydration
   ♦ Tourniquet effect

2. Hyperglobulinaemia can be assocaited with a normal serum total protein level when there is an assocaited hypo-albuminaemia.

Serous fluid albumin (? Transudate, ? Exudate)

Serum [albumin] – Serous fluid [albumin]
>15 g/L = transudate
<15 g/L = exudate

Hyperglobulinaemia

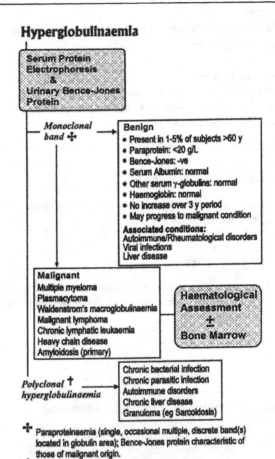

Serum Protein Electrophoresis & Urinary Bence-Jones Protein

Monoclonal band ✠ ⟶ **Benign**
- Present in 1-5% of subjects >60 y
- Paraprotein: <20 g/L
- Bence-Jones: -ve
- Serum Albumin: normal
- Other serum γ-globulins: normal
- Haemoglobin: normal
- No increase over 3 y period
- May progress to malignant condition

Associated conditions:
Autoimmune/Rheumatological disorders
Viral infections
Liver disease

Malignant
Multiple myeloma
Plasmacytoma
Waldenstrom's macroglobulinaemia
Malignant lymphoma
Chronic lymphatic leukaemia
Heavy chain disease
Amyloidosis (primary)

Haematological Assessment ± Bone Marrow

Polyclonal † *hyperglobulinaemia*
Chronic bacterial infection
Chronic parasitic infection
Autoimmune disorders
Chronic liver disease
Granuloma (eg Sarcoidosis)

✠ Paraproteinaemia (single, occasional multiple, discrete band(s) located in globulin area); Bence-Jones protein characteristic of those of malignant origin.

† Diffuse increase in serum gamma-globulins; Bence-Jones protein absent. Oligoclonal band(s) also may be associated with inflammatory response

Evaluation of hyperglobulinaemia

Hypoproteinaemia

Commonest causes
- Hypoalbuminaemia
- Secondary hypoglobulinaemia

Haemodilution
water overload, sample from IV infusion arm

Hypoalbuminaemia *(see Table page 113)*

Hypogammaglobulinaemia
Decreased synthesis
Transient
neonate/infants
Primary
genetically defective immune system *(see page 112)*
Secondary
Haematological disorders: *myeloma, chronic lymphatic leukaemia, lymphosarcoma*
Toxins: *uraemia, corticosteroid therapy, cytotoxic therapy, diabetes mellitus, coeliac disease*
Acquired immune deficiency syndrome
Protein loss
Skin: *burns, exudative lesions*
Gut: *protein-losing enteropathy*
Renal: *nephrotic syndrome*

Miscellaneous
pregnancy (third trimester)

Notes on immunoglobulins

Reference ranges

IgG: Normal adult levels at birth, falls to below 40% of adult levels at 2-4 months, returns to adult levels at 2-3 years.

IgM: Less than 20% of adult levels at birth, reaches adult levels at about nine months of age.

IgA: Very low levels at birth, slow rise to reach adult levels at about fourteen years of age.

Primary immune deficiency: A large variety has been described and includes:

(1) *Severe combined deficiency* (all immunoglobulins): Swiss type, sex-linked form.

(2) *Combined immune deficiency:* associated with (a) thymoma, (b) achondroplasia, (c) thyromocytopenia and eczema.

(3) *Hypogammaglobulinaemia:* X-linked, Burton type.

(4) *Selective deficiencies:* Type I (IgA, IgM), Type II (IgA, IgG), Type III (IgG), Type IV (IgA), Type V (IgM).

Hypoalbuminaemia *(see Figure page 114)*

Commonest causes
  ♦ Liver disease
  ♦ Malnutrition
  ♦ Nephrotic syndrome
  ♦ Acute illness/infection

Haemodilution
  Pregnancy, iv therapy, congestive cardiac failure, cirrhosis, antidiuresis (drugs, SIADH, *see page 6*)
Decreased synthesis
  Deficient precursors: *malabsorption, malnutrition*
  Severe liver disease: *chronic hepatitis, cirrhosis*
  Acute phase reaction
  Analbuminaemia
Altered distribution
  Injury, infection, inflammation
  Malignancy
  Liver failure/cirrhosis
Loss from body
  Skin: *burns, exudative lesions*
  Gut: *protein-losing enteropathy (malignancy, inflammation, mucosal injury)*
  Renal: *nephrotic syndrome*
Increased catabolism
  Malignancy
  Acute phase reaction
Miscellaneous
  Acute/chronic illness
  Malignancy

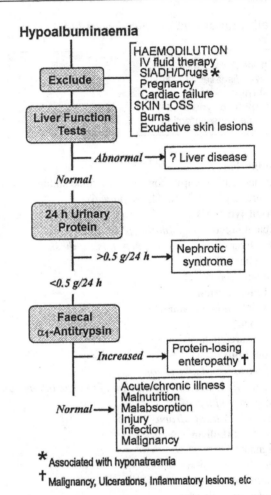

Hypoalbuminaemia

Exclude
- HAEMODILUTION
  - IV fluid therapy
  - SIADH/Drugs *
  - Pregnancy
  - Cardiac failure
- SKIN LOSS
  - Burns
  - Exudative skin lesions

Liver Function Tests

— *Abnormal* → ? Liver disease

Normal

24 h Urinary Protein

— *>0.5 g/24 h* → Nephrotic syndrome

<0.5 g/24 h

Faecal α_1-Antitrypsin

— *Increased* → Protein-losing enteropathy †

Normal → Acute/chronic illness
Malnutrition
Malabsorption
Injury
Infection
Malignancy

* Associated with hyponatraemia

† Malignancy, Ulcerations, Inflammatory lesions, etc

Evaluation of hypoalbuminaemia

15 Lipids

(See pages 119, 120 for Fredrickson classification & clinical aspects)

Predominant hypercholesterolaemia

Approach to evaluation
- ♦ Check fasting lipids + full lipid profile *(page 118)*
- ♦ Exclude secondary causes
- ♦ If primary:
  - ● Family studies including children
  - ● Assess risk factors *(page 117)* & cardiovascular status

Secondary
    Diabetes mellitus
    Hypothyroidism
    Nephrotic syndrome
    Cholestasis/biliary obstruction
    Pregnancy
    Drugs: *thiazide diuretics, β-blockers, oestrogens, cyclosporin*
    Pancreatic disease
    Anorexia nervosa
    Acute intermittent porphyria
    Dysglobulinaemia/myelomatosis

Primary
    Familial combined hyperlipidaemia
    Familial hypercholesterolaemia
    Polygenic (common) hypercholesterolaemia

Predominant hypertriglyceridaemia

Approach to evaluation
 ♦ Check fasting lipid + full lipid profile *(page 118)*
 ♦ Exclude secondary causes

Note
 ● If triglyceride >25 mmol/l treat immediately
 ● Subjects with serum triglycerides >10 mmol/L have a high
    risk of depeloping acute pancreatitis

Secondary
 Pancreatitis
 Hypothyroidism
 Diabetes mellitus (poorly controlled)
 Obesity
 Alcohol excess
 Nephrotic syndrome, Renal failure
 Drugs: *Oestrogens, oral contraceptives, β-blockers, retinoids,*
    corticosteroids
 Systemic lupus erythematosus
 Dysglobulinaemia/myelomatosis
 Gauchers disease, Glycogen storage disease
Primary
 Familial combined hyperlipidaemia
 Fanilial endogenous hypertriglyceridaeamia
 Familial hyperchylomicronaemia: *Lipoprotein lipase*
    deficiency, Apolipoprotein CII deficiency

Mixed hyperlipidaemia

Approach to evaluation
- ◆ Check fasting lipids + full lipid profile *(page 118)*
- ◆ Exclude secondary causes
- ◆ If primary:
  - • Family studies inc children
  - • Assess risk factors *(below)* & cardiovascular status

Secondary
  Diabetes mellitus (poorly controlled)
  Severe hypothyroidism
  Nephrotic syndrome, Renal failure
  Cholestasis/biliary obstruction
  Dysgolbulinaemia/myelomatosis
Primary
  Familial combined hyperlipidaemia
  Dysbetalipoproteinaemia (broad β disease or Type III)
  Hyperapobetalipoproteinaemia

Risk factors: Coronary heart disease
- • Poorly controlled hypertension
- • Poorly controlled diabetes mellitus
- • Obesity (>30% ideal weight)
- • Smoking
- • Male
- • Low HDL-cholesterol
- • Definitive coronary heart disease
- • Family history of premature coronary heart disease

Full lipid profile

Patient preparation

- Fasting 10–14 h prior to test
- No smoking just prior to collection
- Usual diet
- No heavy exercise just prior to collection

Laboratory aspects

Estimate
  Total cholesterol
  Triglycerides
  HDL-cholesterol
  Calculate LDL-cholesterol

If triglycerides >10 mmol/L
  Store serum over night at 4°C
  Inspect for creamy layer & turbidity

Clear serum + creamy surface layer: Chylomicrons

Turbid serum: increased VLDL (Type IV)

Turbid serum + creamy surface layer: Type V, Type III

Fredrickson classification of lipoprotein abnormalities.

Fredrickson Type	Electrophoretic Pattern	Lipoprotein Increase	Cholesterol	Triglyceride
I	↑ Chylomicrons	Chylomicrons	N	↑↑
IIa	↑ β-lipoproteins	LDL	↑↑	N
IIb	↑ β + pre-β-lipoproteins	LDL + VLDL	↑↑	↑
III	Broad β	IDL	↑	↑
IV	↑ pre-β-lipoproteins	VLDL	N-↑↑	↑
V	↑ Chylomicrons & pre-β-lipoproteins	Chylomicrons & VLDL	N-↑	↑

LDL low density lipoprotein, VLDL very low density lipoprotein, IDL intermediate density lipoprotein.

Features of main types of hyperlipidaemias

Type	I	IIa	IIb	III	IV	V
Main chemical abnormality	T	C	C&T	C&T	T	T
Appearance: fasting serum (*after 12 hours at 4°C*)	Creamy surface layer	Clear	Slightly turbid	Turbid, small creamy layer	Turbid	Turbid with creamy layer
Usual age of presentation	Under 10	Any age	Any age	Over 30	Over 20	Over 20
Associated with:						
Cardiovascular disease	No	Yes	Yes	Yes	Probably	Probably not
Abdominal pain/pancreatitis	Yes	No	No	No	Rarely	Yes
Impaired glucose tolerance	No	Yes	Yes	Yes	Yes	Yes
Hyperuricaemia	No	No	No	Yes	Yes	Yes
Xanthoma: Eruptive	+	-	-	-	+	+
Tuberous	-	+	+	+	Rarely	-
Tendinous	-	+	+	+	-	-
Planar	-	Occassionally		+	-	-

T = Raised serum triglyceride; C = Raised serum total cholesterol

16 Thyroid

Low serum TSH *(see Figures pages 122, 123)*

Commonest causes
♦ Thyrotoxicosis
♦ Subclinical toxicosis
♦ Elderly subjects

Euthyroidism *(Normal fT₄)*
  Sick euthyroid *(fT₄ Variable)*
  Pregnancy (first trimester)
  Acute psychiatric illness
  Drugs: *Glucocorticoids, Dopamine, Verapamil, NSAIDs*
  Subclinical hyperthyroidism
  Elderly subjects
  Reference range variant
Hypothyroidism *(Depressed fT₄)*
  Hypopituitarism
  Hypothalamic disease
Hyperthyroidism *(Elevated fT₄)*
  Graves' disease
  Toxic adenoma
  Toxic multinodular goitre
  Trophoblastic tumours
  Thyroiditis: subacute, postpartum, Hashimoto's
  Iodine-induced (Jodbasedow)
  Amiodarone therapy
  T₃-toxicosis *(Normal fT₄)*
  T₄, T₃ medication (iatrogenic, self-abuse)
  Metastatic thyroid malignancy

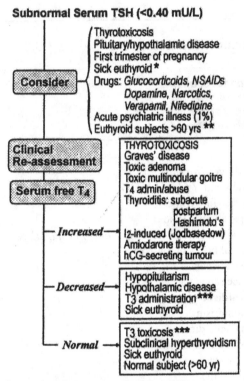

Subnormal Serum TSH (<0.40 mU/L)

Consider
- Thyrotoxicosis
- Pituitary/hypothalamic disease
- First trimester of pregnancy
- Sick euthyroid *
- Drugs: *Glucocorticoids, NSAIDs Dopamine, Narcotics, Verapamil, Nifedipine*
- Acute psychiatric illness (1%)
- Euthyroid subjects >60 yrs **

Clinical Re-assessment

Serum free T4

Increased
THYROTOXICOSIS
- Graves' disease
- Toxic adenoma
- Toxic multinodular goitre
- T4 admin/abuse
- Thyroiditis: subacute postpartum Hashimoto's
- I2-induced (Jodbasedow)
- Amiodarone therapy
- hCG-secreting tumour

Decreased
- Hypopituitarism
- Hypothalamic disease
- T3 administration ***
- Sick euthyroid

Normal
- T3 toxicosis ***
- Subclinical hyperthyroidism
- Sick euthyroid
- Normal subject (>60 yr)

* **Sick Euthyroid:** starvation/calorie deprivation; acute febrile illness, myocardial infarct, acute respiratory failure, surgical operations, renal failure, cirrhosis

** 3-5% of euthyroid subjects >60 yrs have a suppressed serum TSH

***Serum T3 increased

Evaluation of a suppressed TSH *(see list page 121)*

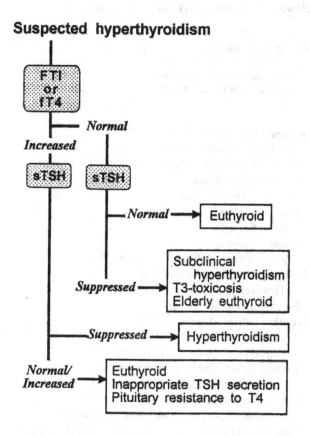

Suspected hyperthyroidism

sTSH sensitive TSH assay, fT4 free T4,
FTI free thyroxine index

Evaluation of suspected hyperthyroidism

Elevated serum TSH *(see Figure page 125)*

Commonest causes
- Primary hypothyroidism
- Subclinicla hypothyroidism
- Reference range variant

Euthyroidism *(Normal fT₄)*
  Subclinical hypothyroidism
  Recovery from sick euthyroid
  Acute psychiatric illness
  Reference range variant
  Elderly subjects
  Lithium therapy
  Iodine deficiency
  T_4/T_3-resistant syndromes *(Elevated fT₄)*
Hyperthyroidism *(Elevated fT₄)*
  TSH-secreting tumour
  Pituitary resistance to T_4/T_3
Hypothyroidism *(Depressed fT₄)*
  Primary hypothyroidism: congenital (Cretinism),
      Hashimoto's, ablative, idiopathic
  Enzyme defects (dyshormonogenesis)
  Iodine deficiency
  Goitrogens/antithyroid drugs
  Thyroiditis (hypo-phase): subacute, postpartum
  Lithium therapy
  Amiodarone therapy
  Peripheral resistance to T_4/T_3 *(Elevated fT₄)*

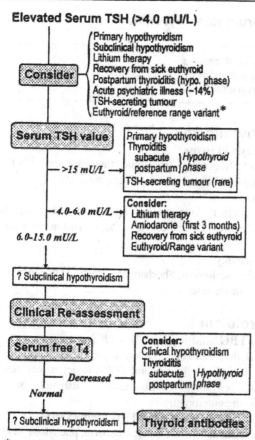

Elevated Serum TSH (>4.0 mU/L)

Consider
- Primary hypothyroidism
- Subclinical hypothyroidism
- Lithium therapy
- Recovery from sick euthyroid
- Postpartum thyroiditis (hypo. phase)
- Acute psychiatric illness (~14%)
- TSH-secreting tumour
- Euthyroid/reference range variant *

Serum TSH value

>15 mU/L →
- Primary hypothyroidism
- Thyroiditis
  - subacute } Hypothyroid
  - postpartum } phase
- TSH-secreting tumour (rare)

4.0-6.0 mU/L →
Consider:
- Lithium therapy
- Amiodarone (first 3 months)
- Recovery from sick euthyroid
- Euthyroid/Range variant

6.0-15.0 mU/L

? Subclinical hypothyroidism

Clinical Re-assessment

Serum free T4

Decreased →
Consider:
- Clinical hypothyroidism
- Thyroiditis
  - subacute } Hypothyroid
  - postpartum } phase

Normal

? Subclinical hypothyroidism → **Thyroid antibodies**

* Around 2% of elderly have an elevated TSH. Upper reference limit is difficult to define--skewed distribution and outliers are common--value lies between 3.0-6.0 mU/L.

Evaluation of an Elevated TSH *(see list page 124)*

Low serum total thyroxine

Commonest causes
- ◆ Hypothyroidism
- ◆ Drug effects

Hypothyroidism

Loss of thyroid tissue
Idiopathic; Dysgenesis; Iatrogenic: thyroidectomy, ^{131}I therapy;
Thyroiditis: Hashimoto's, postpartum, subacute

Goitrous
Synthesis defect; Autoimmune: Hashimoto's disease; Dietary:
iodine deficiency; Drugs: carbimazole, propylthiouracil, lithium,
iodine

TSH deficiency
Pituitary disease: tumour, Shechan's syndrome; Deficiency of TRH:
hypothalamic disease

Euthyroidism

Reduced TBG binding sites *(Low TBG states)*
Congenital; drugs: androgen therapy, asparaginase, corticosteroids;
Disease (including albumin and TBPA deficiencies): nephrotic
syndrome, cirrhosis, malnutrition, Cushing's syndrome,
protein-losing enteropathy

Hormone displacement from TBG binding sites
salicylates, free fatty acids (oleic), heparin, phenytoin, diazepam,
frusemide (high dose)

Drugs that increase hormone metabolism
phenobarbital, phenytoin, carbamazepine

Altered hormone metabolism
severe non-thyroid illness; thyroxine replacement therapy (low T_3)

High serum total thyroxine

Commonest causes
- Thyrotoxicosis
- Increased thyroxine binding globulin (TBG)

Hyperthyroidism
Thyroid overactivity
Grave's disease, Toxic multinodular goitre, Toxic adenoma, TSH-secreting tumour (rare), T_3 toxicosis
Thyroid destruction
Subacute thyroiditis (acute phase), Hashimoto's disease (acute phase)
Ectopic thyroid
Stroma ovarii (rare), Metastatic thyroid carcinoma (rare)
Exogenous thyroxine
Thyrotoxicosis factitia, Iatrogenic
Drugs
Amiodarone (sometimes)
Euthyroidism
Increased thyroxine-binding globulin
Congenital, Pregnancy, Oestrogen therapy (oral contraceptives)
Increased thyroxine binding by albumin or prealbumin
Familial dysalbuminaemic hyperthyroxinaemia
Peripheral resistance to thyroid hormones
Reketoff's syndrome, Selective pituitary resistance
Acute non-thyroidal illness
Medical illness, Psychiatric illness, Hyperemesis gravidarum
Antibodies to thyroid hormones
Drugs
Amiodarone, Iopanoic acid, Propanolol, Amphetamines

17 Adrenal cortex

Hypercortisolism *(see Figure page 129)*

> ### Common causes of Cushing's syndrome
> ♦ **ACTH-dependent** (75%)
>   Cushing's disease (60%):
>   Pituitary adenoma *
>   Pituitary Hyperplasia*
>   Ectopic-ACTH (15%)
> ♦ **ACTH-independent** (25%)
>   Carcinoma (15%), Adenoma (10%)
> (*Pituitary causes: ~90% adenoma, ~10% hyperplasia)

Physiological
   Stress, Obesity, Depression
Excess ACTH production
   Pituitary disease: *Cushing's disease*
   Hypothalamic disease: *excess CRF production*
   Ectopic ACTH: Malignancy (lung, thymus, pancreas, ovary)
Excess cortisol (Pituitary-independent)
   Adrenal tumour: *adenoma, carcinoma*
   Alcoholism
   Iatrogenic: *steroid therapy*
Excess cortisol-binding globulin
   Oestrogen therapy; Pregnancy

> **Intermittent Cushing's syndrome:** Cushing's syndrome can present in a cyclic manner, ie, characteristic clinical features but with periods of normal cortisol secretion rate resulting in normal screening tests. The only approach to this problem is persistent investigation& serial estimations of urinary free cortisol.

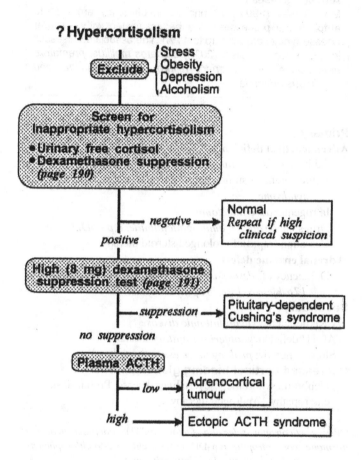

Evaluation of suspected Cushing's syndrome.

Hypocortisolism   *(see Figure page 131)*

> **Addison's disease**
> Most cases (>90%) of primary insufficiency are due to autoimmune processes. May be associated with a similar disease in other organs (up to 41%). The associated diseases include *hypothyroidism (20%), diabetes mellitus, premature menopause and ovarian failure, hypopituitarism, and pernicious anaemia*

Primary
Adrenocortical deficiency

    Addison's disease: *autoimmune, tuberculosis*

    Acute adrenal insufficiency: *Waterhouse-Friederichson*
        syndrome

    Iatrogenic: *adrenalectomy*

    Drugs: *metyrapone, aminoglutethimide, o,p'-DDD*

    Cessation (rapid)of prolonged steroid therapy

Adrenal enzyme defects

    Deficiency of: *desmolase, 3β-hydroxysteroid dehydrogenase,*
        17α-hydroxylase, 11β-hydroxylase

Secondary

    CRF deficiency: *hypothalamic disease*

    ACTH deficiency: *anterior pituitary disease*

    Steroid therapy: *prolonged/excessive* (withdrawl)

Decreased cortisol-binding globulin

    Nephrotic syndrome; Severe liver disease; Protein-losing
    enteropathy; Androgen therapy

CRF: *corticotropin releasing factor;* ACTH: *adrenocorticotropic hormone (corticotropin);* o,p'-DDD: *1,1-dichloro-2-(o-chlorophenyl)-2-(p- chlorophenyl) ethane (Lysodren, mitotane)*

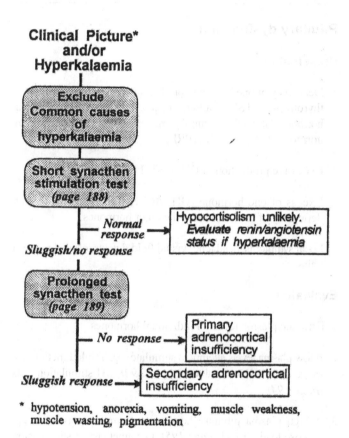

Clinical Picture*
and/or
Hyperkalaemia

Exclude Common causes of hyperkalaemia

Short synacthen stimulation test *(page 188)*

Normal response → Hypocortisolism unlikely. *Evaluate renin/angiotensin status if hyperkalaemia*

Sluggish/no response

Prolonged synacthen test *(page 189)*

No response → Primary adrenocortical insufficiency

Sluggish response → Secondary adrenocortical insufficiency

* hypotension, anorexia, vomiting, muscle weakness, muscle wasting, pigmentation

Evaluation of suspected hypocortisolism

18 Anterior pituitary

Pituitary dysfunction

Presentation

1. Deficiency of one, or some, or all anterior pituitary hormones - thyrotropin (TSH), adrenocorticotropin (ACTH), growth hormone (GH), follicle stimula-ting hormone (FSH), luteinizing hormone (LH), prolactin (PRL).

2. Excessive production of GH, ACTH or PRL

3. Excess of one hormone (GH, ACTH, PRL) associated with deficiency of one or more of the other hormones.

4. Local symptoms: headache, visual field defects, cranial nerve II palsy

Evaluation

1. Estimate plasma levels of individual hormones

2. If low plasma levels attempt to stimulate, eg, Triple function test *(page 192)*, TRH-stimulation *(page 192)*, GH-stimulation tests *(page 194)*

3. If high plasma pituitary hormones attempt suppression, eg, glucose load for GH *(page 195)*, Dexamethasone suppression test for ACTH *(page 190)*

5. Imaging, eg, MRI, CAT scan for suspected tumours.

Hypopituitarism

Multiple deficiencies
Tumour/pituitary: adenoma, secondary deposits
Tumour/hypothalamic: craniopharyngioma, meningioma, glioma,
   lymphoma, leukaemia, secondary deposits e.g. breast
Infarction (apoplexy): Postpartum - Sheehan's syndrome;
   Vascular disease - atherosclerosis
Granuloma: sarcoidosis, histiocytosis X
Trauma: head injury
Infection: tuberculosis, abscess, syphilis
Autoimmune: lymphocytic hypophysitis
Iatrogenic: surgery, irradiation
Haemochromatosis
Amyloidosis
Hypothalamic disease: tumour, trauma, infection, cyst,
   degenerative

Isolated deficiencies *(congenital)*
Hypothalamic: TRH, CRF
Pituitary: GH, ACTH, TSH, Gonadotropins

Hyperpituitarism

Growth hormone: adenoma (Acromegaly, giantism) - *page 195*
Corticotropin : adenoma (Cushing's disease) - *pages 129, 190*
Prolactin: hyperprolactinaemia *(see page 138)*
Thyrotropin: adenoma (Thyrotoxicosis - rare)

19 Reproductive system

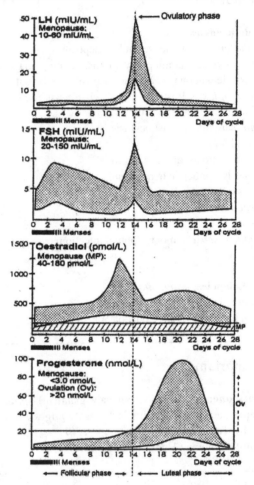

Normal menstrual cycle: Plasma hormones

Detectable (>25 mIU/mL): 8 days post ovulation
9 days post midcycle
1 day post implantation

Rise: doubles every 2-3 days (mean 2.7 days)

Gestational age   mIU/mL

0-1 week	0-50
1-2 weeks	50-500
2-3 weeks	100-5,000
3-4 weeks	500-10,000
4-5 weeks	1,000-50,000
5-6 weeks	10,000-100,000
6-8 weeks	15,000-200,000
8-12 weeks	10,000-100,000
2nd trimester	3,000-50,000
3rd trimester	1,000-20,000

Half-life (t1/2): 32-37 h (mean 36 h)

Ectopic/Abortion

48h observation: Increase <66% suggests ectopic
False +ve 15%
False -ve 13%

Doubling time >7 days suggests ectopic

Falling values: t1/2 <1.4 days = complete abortion
t1/2 >7 days = ectopic

Uterine gestational sac visible ultrasonically
Transvaginal: ~1000 mIU/mL
Transabdominal: ~2000 mIU/mL

Pregnancy/ectopic/abortion and serum hCG levels

Amenorrhoea   *(see Figure page 137)*

Commonest causes
- ◆ Pregnancy, Menopause
- ◆ Hypothalamic: 65%–75%
- ◆ Pituitary (prolactinoma): ~20%

Pregnancy, Menopause

Hypothalamic: Psychological stress/depression
Anorexia nervosa/bulimia/starvation
Severe exercise/weight loss
Chronic disease
Thyroid disease
Post-oral contraceptive amenorrhoea.
Hypothalamic disease (tumours, etc)

Pituitary: Prolactinoma/hyperprolactinaemia *(page 138)*
Hypopituitarism
Acromegaly
Cushing's disease

Ovary: *Premature ovarian failure*
Chromosomal abnormalities
Autoimmune disease
Infections
Familial
Iatrogenic (chemotherapy, irradiation, etc)
Hyperandrogenic
Polycystic ovarian disease
Hyperthecosis
Neoplasia (Sertoli-Leydig tumours, lipoid cell)

Uterus: Malformations, Dysgenesis, Atrophic disease

Amenorrhoea

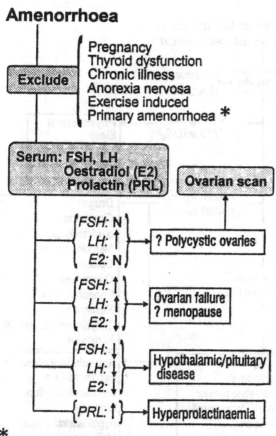

Exclude
- Pregnancy
- Thyroid dysfunction
- Chronic illness
- Anorexia nervosa
- Exercise induced
- Primary amenorrhoea *

Serum: FSH, LH
Oestradiol (E2)
Prolactin (PRL)

Ovarian scan

FSH: N
LH: ↑
E2: N
→ ? Polycystic ovaries

FSH: ↑
LH: ↑
E2: ↓
→ Ovarian failure ? menopause

FSH: ↓
LH: ↓
E2: ↓
→ Hypothalamic/pituitary disease

PRL: ↑
→ Hyperprolactinaemia

* Chromosome abnormalities and ovarian failure are more common in women who have never had a spontaneous period.

Evaluation of amenorrhoea

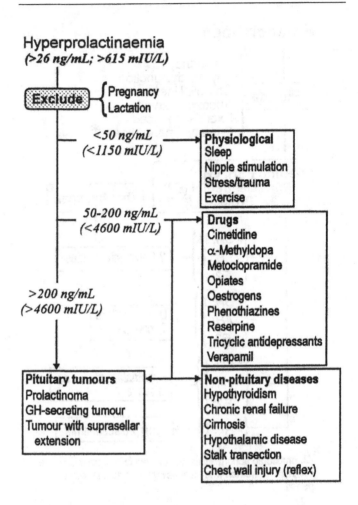

Hyperprolactinaemia

Infertility in the female *(see Figure page 140)*

Commonest causes
- ◆ Pelvic disease: ~25%
- ◆ Anovulation: ~30%
- ◆ Luteal phase dysfunction: 10%–15%
- NB ▪ 10%–15% of couples infertile
  - ▪ ~40% due to male partner

Anovulation
Pituitary   }
Hypothalamic   } *see Table page 136*
Ovarian   }
Adrenal: Cushing's syndrome, enzyme defects
Thyroid: Hyper- & hypothyroidism
Diabetes mellitus

Luteal phase dysfunction *(<10 days, peak plasma progesterone <30 nmol/L)*
    Hyperprolactinaemia
    Extremes of reproductive life
    Severe exercise
    Excessive weight loss
    Idiopathic

Pelvic disease
    Tubal disease: obstruction, etc
    Uterine disease: endometriosis, infection, etc
    Cervical disease.

Infertility (♀)

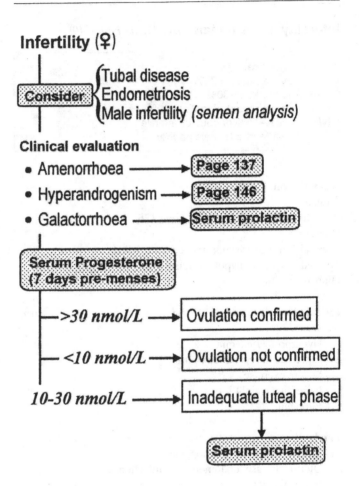

Consider {Tubal disease, Endometriosis, Male infertility *(semen analysis)*}

Clinical evaluation

- Amenorrhoea ⟶ Page 137
- Hyperandrogenism ⟶ Page 146
- Galactorrhoea ⟶ Serum prolactin

Serum Progesterone (7 days pre-menses)

— >30 nmol/L ⟶ Ovulation confirmed

— <10 nmol/L ⟶ Ovulation not confirmed

10-30 nmol/L ⟶ Inadequate luteal phase ⟶ Serum prolactin

Evaluation of infertility in the female

Male infertility *(see Figure page 142)*

Commonest causes
- ♦ Seminiferous tubule failure: 50%–60%
- ♦ Varicocele: ~20%
- ♦ Obstructed vas deferens: ~10%
- ♦ Endocrine dysfunction: <10%

NB Male infertility is main problem in ~40% of couples

Hypothalamic/pituitary
  Idiopathic
  Tumours
  Hyperprolactinaemia
Primary testicular disorders
  Klinefelter's syndrome
  Cryptorchidism
  Orchitis
  Irradiation
  Cytotoxic therapy
Idiopathic seminiferous tubule failure
  Azospermia, oligospermia
  Poor sperm motility
Obstructed vas deferens
Varicocele
Chronic disease

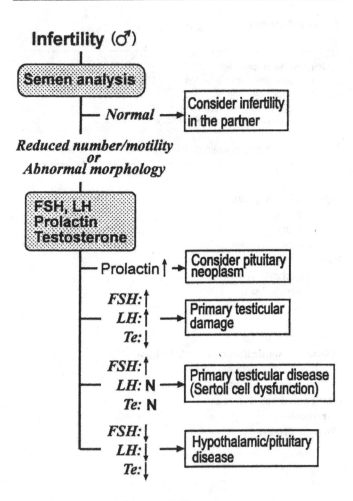

Evaluation of male infertility

Male hypogonadism *(see Figure page 144)*

Delayed puberty
Hypogonadotrophic hypogonadism *(Low/normal FSH, LH)*
    Constitutional (temporary) delay
    Prader-Willi Syndrome
    Laurence-Moon-Biedel Syndrome
    Kallmann's syndrome
    Hypopituitarism
Hypergonadotrophic Hypogonadism *(High FSH, LH)*
    Klienfelter's syndrome
    Bilateral anorchia
    Gonadal dysgenesis
    Testicular disease: *autoimmune, infection, irradiation,*
        chemotherapy
    Androgen insensitivity

Postpubertal hypogonadism
Hypogonadotrophic hypogonadism *(Low/normal FSH, LH)*
    Chronic illness, Malnutrition
    Cushing's syndrome
    Hyperprolactinaemia
    Hypothyroidism
    Hypopituitarism
    Haemochromatosis
    Drugs: *Alcohol, Spironolactone*
    Idiopathic
Hypergonadotrophic hypogonadism *(High FSH, LH)*
    Idiopathic
    Klienfelter's syndrome
    Testicular disease: *trauma, infiltrations, infection,*
        chemotherapy, radiotherapy
    Elderly men (male climacteric)

? Hypogonadism (Male)
(? hypoandrogenism)

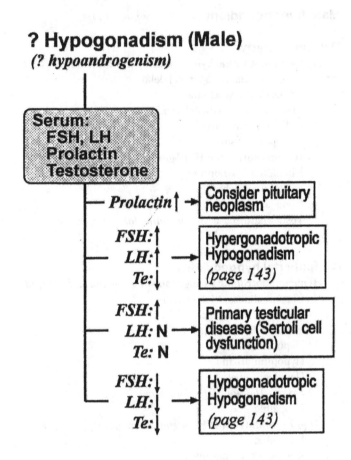

Serum:
FSH, LH
Prolactin
Testosterone

— Prolactin↑ → Consider pituitary neoplasm

FSH:↑
— LH:↑ → Hypergonadotropic Hypogonadism
Te:↓ *(page 143)*

FSH:↑
— LH: N → Primary testicular disease (Sertoli cell dysfunction)
Te: N

FSH:↓
— LH:↓ → Hypogonadotropic Hypogonadism
Te:↓ *(page 143)*

Evaluation of hypogonadism in the male

Hirsutism and virilization *(see Figure page 146)*

Commonest causes
* Non-androgenic
   Racial/familial
   Drug-related
* Polycystic ovarian disease
NB Virilism suggests serious disorder — consider tumour

Non androgenic
Racial/Familial; Menopause; Endocrine: *hypothyroidism, acromegaly, hyperprolactinaemia*; Drugs: *Glucocorticoids, Phenytoin, Diazoxide,*; Porphyria

Androgenic
Adrenal
   Congenital adrenal hyperpalsia: 21 & *11-β hydroxylase deficiency*
   Tumour: *adenoma, carcinoma*
   Cushing's syndrome
Ovary
   Polycystic ovarian disease (PCOD)
   Hyperthecosis
   Tumour: *Sertoli-Leydig cell, dysgerminoma, lipoid cell*
   Intersex (ovotestis)
Exogenous
   Androgens; Danazol; Progestational agents
Idiopathic
   Increased 5-α-reductase activity

Hirsutism/virilization

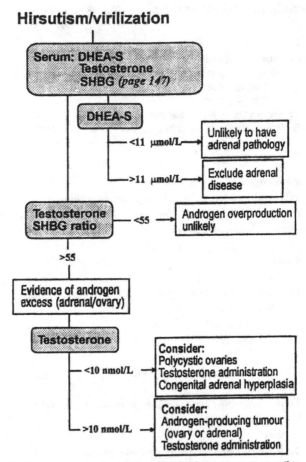

SHBG: sex hormone-binding globulin   DHEA-S: dehydroepiandrosterone sulfate

Evaluation of hirsutism & hyperandrogenism

Sex hormone-binding globulins (SHBG)

Increased Serum SHBG
  Oestrogen Excess
    Pregnancy
    Exogenous
    Oral contraceptive medication
    Cirrhosis (males)
  Drugs: *Phenytoin, Carbamazepine, Thyroxine*
  Thyrotoxicosis
  Hypogonadism (males)
  Anorexia nervosa
  Fasting/Starvation

Decreased Serum SHBG
  Hyperandrogenism
    Endogenous
    Exogenous
  Obesity
  Hyperinsulinism
  Hypothyroidism
  Acromegaly
  Hyperprolactinaemia
  Nephrotic syndrome
  Drugs: *Androgens, Danazol, Progestational agents*

20 Iron

Serum ferritin

Low serum levels: Values <12 µg/L indicate iron deficiency;
values >100 µg/L are unlikely in iron deficiency; values between
12 & 100 µg/L are equivocal but possible in iron deficiency.
High serum values: Values above the upper reference limit
may be due to two conditions:
 ♦ Iron overload
 ♦ Release from cell stores: infection, malignancy, infarction

Low serum ferritin
Iron deficiency

High serum ferritin
A. Iron overload *(see Table page 152)*
B. Iron stores not increased*
Acute phase reactions
Chronic disease
Liver disease: *Alcoholic, Chronic active hepatitis, Acute
 hepatitis, Fatty infiltration, Secondary malignancy*
Renal disease: *Acute and chronic failure, Dialysis*
HIV infection
Non-HIV infections: *Sepsis, Pneumonia, Colitis,
 Tuberculosis, Cytomegalovirus*
Malignancy: *Prostate, Lung, Colon, Liver, Lymphoma,
 Myeloma, Leukaemia*
Still's disease

* *A number of these non-iron overload disorders have been
associated with values >1000 µg/L, some up to 5000 mg/L.*

Low serum iron *(see Figure page 150)*

> **Factors affecting serum iron level**
> * *Age:* Lower levels during first two years of life.
> * *Sex:* Levels 10-20% lower in females.
> * *Time:* The circadian rhythm may vary up to 50% (highest in morning, 8 to 10 AM, lowest at 9 PM).
> * *Pregnancy:* Elevated during first trimester
> * *Menses:* Levels fall just before and during first day of menses.
> * *Diet:* A diet high in iron (or medication) results in transient high values.

Physiological
Pre-menstrual state
Biological variation

Iron deficiency
Low intake: *nutritional*
Increased requirement: *growth, pregnancy, lactation; therapy of pernicious anaemia*
Increased loss: *acute/chronic haemorrhage*

Low transferrin level
Infection: acute, chronic
Collagen diseases
Malignancy
Renal failure
Protein-losing states: *nephrosis, protein-losing enteropathy*
Atransferrinaemia

Iron deficiency

Causes: *see page 149*

Characteristics: Sequence of events to anaemia are —

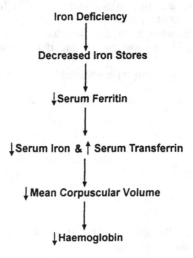

Evaluation: *(see Figure page 151)*

Blood picture: hypochromic microcytic anaemia
Mild anisocytosis
Iron studies: Low serum iron
High serum transferrin
Low saturation of transferrin
Low serum Ferritin

Microcytic anaemia (MCV <78 fL)

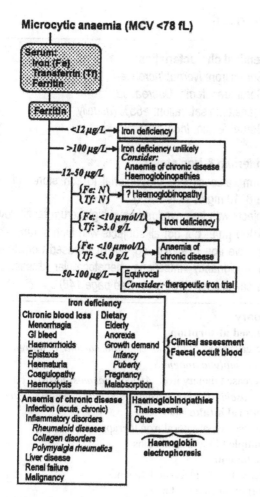

Serum:
Iron (Fe)
Transferrin (Tf)
Ferritin

Ferritin

— *<12 μg/L* → Iron deficiency

— *>100 μg/L* → Iron deficiency unlikely
Consider:
Anaemia of chronic disease
Haemoglobinopathies

— *12-50 μg/L*

{ Fe: N
  Tf: N } → ? Haemoglobinopathy

{ Fe: <10 μmol/L
  Tf: >3.0 g/L } → Iron deficiency

{ Fe: <10 μmol/L
  Tf: <3.0 g/L } → Anaemia of chronic disease

— *50-100 μg/L* → Equivocal
Consider: therapeutic iron trial

Iron deficiency		
Chronic blood loss	**Dietary**	
Menorrhagia	Elderly	
GI bleed	Anorexia	
Haemorrhoids	Growth demand	} Clinical assessment
Epistaxis	*Infancy*	} Faecal occult blood
Haematuria	Puberty	
Coagulopathy	Pregnancy	
Haemoptysis	Malabsorption	

Anaemia of chronic disease	Haemoglobinopathies
Infection (acute, chronic)	Thalassaemia
Inflammatory disorders	Other
Rheumatoid diseases	
Collagen disorders	Haemoglobin
Polymyalgia rheumatica	electrophoresis
Liver disease	
Renal failure	
Malignancy	

Evaluation of iron deficiency

Iron overload

Biochemical characteristics
 ♦ Serum iron: *Normal/Increased*
 ♦ Serun transferrin: *Decreased*
 ♦ Transferrin saturation: *>65% (usually >80%)*
 ♦ Serum ferritin: *Increased*

Serum ferritin & iron stores
 Serum value directly proportional to iron stores (1 µg/L reflects 8–10 mg of stored iron)
 Subjects with iron overload have high serum ferritin levels, eg, >1000 µg/L, but not all subjects with high serum ferritin values have iron overload, eg, ferritin released from tissues during malignancy, infections, hepatocellular disease, etc (values can exceed 5000 µg/L, *see page 148*)

Secondary
  Increased absorption
      Increased red cell turnover: *thalassaemia, acquired haemolytic anaemia*
      Increased dietary iron: *African haemosiderosis, Kaschin-Beck syndrome, alcoholic cirrhosis, iatrogenic*
  Parenteral intake
      Excessive parenteral iron therapy
      Multiple blood transfusions
  Miscellaneous
      Hereditary transferrin deficiency
      Porphyria cutanea tarda
      Sideroblastic anaemia

21 Hypertension

Elevated blood pressure *(see Figure page 155)*

Definition: Chronic elevation of blood pressure to greater
than 140/90 mmHg

Commonest causes
- 90–95% Essential hypertension
- 1–5% Renal hypertension
- <1% Endocrine causes

Primary

Idiopathic (essential): *benign, malignant, low renin, high renin*

Secondary

Renal: parenchymal disease, renovascular

Adrenal medulla: phaeochromocytoma

Adrenal cortex: primary hyperaldosteronism, Cushing's
syndrome, 11-hydroxylase defect, 17-hydroxylase defect,
pseudohyperaldosteronism *(see also page 48)*

Thyroid: thyrotoxicosis

Miscellaneous: coarctation of aorta, toxaemia of pregnancy,
renin-producing tumour, oral contraceptives, licorice
derivatives, mineralocorticoid therapy

Disorders associated with a high incidence of essential hypertension

Diabetes mellitus
Obesity
Hyperparathyroidism
Hyperlipidaemia
Hyperuricaemia

Consider secondary causes if:

- Onset before 40-years or after 55-years

- Marked elevation of blood pressure

- Poor response to accepted antihypertensive therapy

- Abdominal bruit (renovascular)

- Hypokalaemia (aldosteronism)

- Variable pressure with tachycardia and sweating (phaeochromocytoma)

- Decreased femoral pulses (coarctation of aorta)

Hypertension

Routine biochemical evaluation
{ Plasma electrolytes creatinine/urea lipids/urate/calcium

Plasma [creatinine]

RENAL HYPERTENSION
Renovascular disease
Unilateral renal disease
Bilateral renal disease
HYPERTENSIVE RENAL DISEASE

— *High* →

Normal/ mild increase

Plasma [K]

— *Low* —

Exclude: Diuretic therapy
Evaluate: Aldosterone & Renin Status

Normal

Clinical Evaluation

? Essential hypertension
? Mineralocorticoid excess
? Phaeochromocytoma
? Renovascular disease

Evaluate: (1) Catecholamines
(2) Aldosterone & Renin Status
Renal arteriography

Evaluation of hypertension

22 Diarrhoea

Diarrhoea

> **Definition:**   Frequent passage of unformed stools (>200
> g/day) due to excessive stool water
>
> **Classification:** Based on faecal osmolar gap *(page 157)*
>   ♦ Secretory: normal gap
>   ♦ Osmotic: high gap

Secretory diarrhoea *(normal faecal osmolar gap)*
Infectious
Bacteria: salmonella, shigella, cholera, E. coli, clostridia,
          staphylococcus
Parasites: E. histolytica
Non-infectious
Humoral: VIPoma, carcinoid syndrome, Zollinger-Ellison
          syndrome, laxative abuse
Damage to gut wall: enteritis, ulcerative colitis
Villous adenoma of colon
Chloride diarrhoea

Osmotic diarrhoea *(high faecal osmolar gap)*
Overload
 Laxatives e.g. magnesium sulphate
 Poorly absorbable saccharides, e.g. sorbitol, lactulose
Malabsorption
 Carbohydrate, fat, protein
Maldigestion
 Lactase/maltase/sucrase/lipase deficiency

Faecal osmolality and osmolar gap

The osmolal gap of the diarrhoeal fluid is calculated from the following equation:

Osmolar gap = Measured osmolality - calculated osmolality
(mmol/kg)   (mmol/kg)   (mmol/L)

where calculated osmolality = 2 x {[Na] + [K]} (mmol/L)

In *secretory diarrhoea* the measured osmolality is similar to the calculated osmolality (or less than 10 mmol/kg above the calculated osmolality). Often the osmolal gap is negative (calculated osmolality greater than the measured osmolality). This is due to the presence in the diarrhoeal fluid of multivalent anions, i.e. the calculated osmolality assumes that each sodium or potassium ion is balanced by one univalent anion, but complex anions (e.g. PO_4^{3-}, SO_4^{2-}) may be present and this will result in an overestimation of the calculated osmolality.

In *osmotic diarrhoea* the measured osmolality is higher than the calculated osmolality (high gap, eg >20 mmol/kg) due to the presence of osmotically active particles other than sodium and potassium, eg, sugars, fatty acids, organic acids.

23 Coma

Coma *(see Figure page 160)*

> **Common causes**
> - trauma,
> - drug/alcohol overdose,
> - diabetic/hypoglycaemic coma
> - cerebral lesions (stroke, subarachnoid haemorrhage)

Intracerebral pathology

Trauma/Head injury
Infections: encephalitis, meningitis
Haemorrhage: intra-cerebral, subarachnoid, subdural
Space-occupying lesions: tumour, abscess, haematoma, cyst

Intoxications

Alcohol: ethanol, methanol
Narcotics: morphine, pethidine, heroin
Antidepressants: tricyclics, MAO inhibitors
Sedatives/tranquillisers: barbiturates, diazepam, chlorpropamine
Heavy metals: lead, mercury, manganese
Carbon dioxide
Carbon monoxide

Metabolic

Anoxia: cardiac arrest, circulatory collapse, respiratory disorders
Endocrine: hypopituitary coma, adrenal failure, steroid toxicity,
.... *Cont'd next page*

(endocrinc causes of coma cont'd)
　　　　myxocdema coma, hyperthyroid crisis, hyper- and
　　　　hypoparathyroidism, hypoglycaemia, hypergly-
　　　　caemia
Renal failure
Hepatic failure
Electrolytes: 　hypo- and hypernatraemia; hyper- and
　　　　hypocalcaemia
Acid-base: alkalaemia (severe); acidaemia (severe)
Hyperammoniaemia

Miscellaneous

Epilepsy
Hysteria
Hypertensive enccphalopathy
Hypothermia & hyperthermia
Acute porphyria

Degrees of altered mentation

Confusion: Lack of clarity in thinking and inattentiveness.

Stupor: Responsive only to vigorous stimuli.

Coma: unresponsive to any stimuli.

Coma

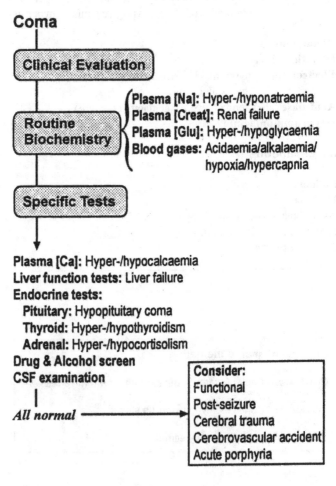

Clinical Evaluation

Routine Biochemistry

Plasma [Na]: Hyper-/hyponatraemia
Plasma [Creat]: Renal failure
Plasma [Glu]: Hyper-/hypoglycaemia
Blood gases: Acidaemia/alkalaemia/
            hypoxia/hypercapnia

Specific Tests

Plasma [Ca]: Hyper-/hypocalcaemia
Liver function tests: Liver failure
Endocrine tests:
    Pituitary: Hypopituitary coma
    Thyroid: Hyper-/hypothyroidism
    Adrenal: Hyper-/hypocortisolism
Drug & Alcohol screen
CSF examination

All normal

Consider:
Functional
Post-seizure
Cerebral trauma
Cerebrovascular accident
Acute porphyria

Evaluation of Coma

24 Polyuria

Polyuria *(see Figures page 162 & 163, dehydration test page 197)*

> **Definition:** daily urine output in excess of three litres.
> **Commonest causes**
> ♦ Diabetes mellitus
> ♦ Functional/psychological over drinking
> ♦ Diuretics & other medications, eg, lithium

Water diuresis

Decreased ADH secretion
Physiological: *compulsive water drinking*
Pathological: *neurogenic diabetes insipidus*

Defective ADH action (nephrogenic diabetes insipidus)
Congenital
Acquired
Renal disease: *pyelonephritis, amyloid, myeloma, polycystic kidney, obstructive uropathy, analgesic nephropathy, interstitial nephritis*
Electrolyte disorders: *hypokalaemia, hypercalcaemia;*
Drugs: *lithium, demeclocycline, methylfluorane*

Solute diuresis

Sodium
Increased intake: *dietary, iatrogenic*
Increased renal loss: *diuretic therapy, renal salt-losing nephritis, renal tubular acidosis, mineralocorticoid deficiency* .... *Cont'd next page*

(solute diuresis cont'd)
Urea
  Increased production: *hypercatabolic states*
  Renal disease: *chronic renal failure, post-obstruction, post-acute tubular necrosis*
Glucose
  Diabetes mellitus
Other solutes e.g. mannitol

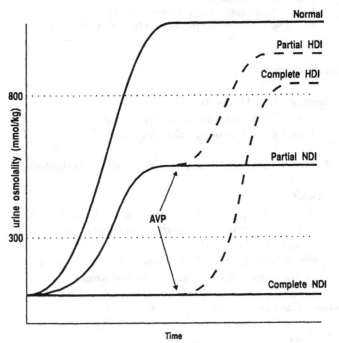

HDI hypothalamic diabetes insipidus, NDI nephrogenic diabetes insipidus

Urinary response to dehydration and Arginine vasopressin *(see page 197)*

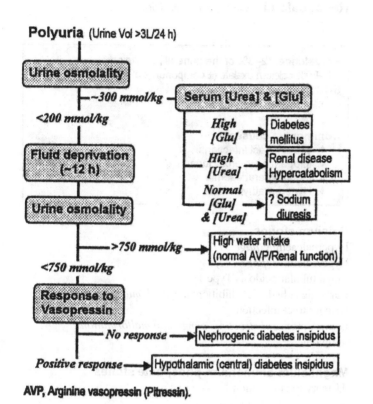

Polyuria (Urine Vol >3L/24 h)

- Urine osmolality
  - ~300 mmol/kg → Serum [Urea] & [Glu]
    - High [Glu] → Diabetes mellitus
    - High [Urea] → Renal disease Hypercatabolism
    - Normal [Glu] & [Urea] → ? Sodium diuresis
  - <200 mmol/kg
    - Fluid deprivation (~12 h)
    - Urine osmolality
      - >750 mmol/kg → High water intake (normal AVP/Renal function)
      - <750 mmol/kg
        - Response to Vasopressin
          - No response → Nephrogenic diabetes insipidus
          - Positive response → Hypothalamic (central) diabetes insipidus

AVP, Arginine vasopressin (Pitressin).

Evaluation of polyuria *(see page 197 for detail, and page 162 for response to AVP)*

25 Nephrolithiasis

Renal calculi *(see Figure page 166)*

Prevalence: 2–3% of the general population
70–80% calcium oxalate (± components of calcium phosphate)
5-10% uric acid
<1% cystine, xanthine

Commonest causes
♦ Urinary tract infections
♦ Idiopathic hypercalciuria
♦ Gout/hyperuricaemia
♦ Hyperparathyroidism

Calcium stones
Hypercalcaemia *(page 51)*
Hypercalciuria *(page 165)*
Renal tubular acidosis Type 1
Carbonic anhydrase inhibition: *acetazolamide*
Urinary tract infection
Urinary stasis: *obstruction, congenital malformations*
Idiopathic

Magnesium-ammonium-phosphate stones
Urinary tract infection

Uric acid stones
Hyperuricosuria: *gout, secondary hyperuricaemia (page 71)*
Low urine output: *obstruction, hot climates*
Idiopathic
.... *Cont'd next page*

(renal calculi cont'd)

Oxalate stones
Hyperoxaluria: *Primary; Secondary: dietary, intestinal disease (Crohn's, gut resection) Idiopathic*

Cystine stones
Cystinuria

Xanthine stones
Xanthinuria
Allopurinol therapy

Causes of hypercalciuria

Hypercalcaemia *(see page 51)*
Primary hyperparathyroidism, Malignancy, Multiple myeloma, Vitamin D excess, Sarcoidosis,Milk-alkali syndrome, Immobilisation

Normocalcaemia
Malignancy, Immobilisation, Hyperthyroidism, Osteoporosis *(senile, postmenopausal)*, steroid therapy, Cushing's syndrome, renal tubular acidosis (Types 1 and 2), Paget's disease, Increased oral calcium intake

Idiopathic hypercalciuria
? Increased gut absorption, ? decreased renal reabsorption, ? excessive bone mobilisation

---

Nephrolithiasis

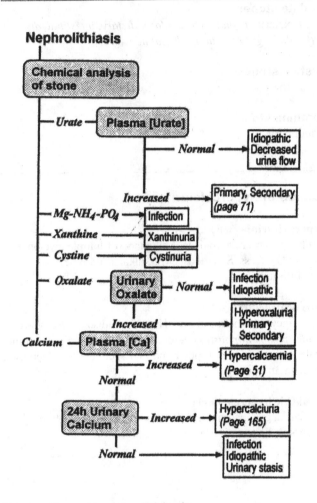

Evaluation of nephrolithiasis

26 Steatorrhoea

Steatorrhoea/malabsorption *(see Figure page168)*

Commonest causes
 ♦ Coeliac disease
 ♦ Tropical sprue
 ♦ Infiltrations of small gut (lymphoma)

Hepato-biliary disease
Cholestasis, Chronic liver disease

Pancreatic disease
Cystic fibrosis, Chronic pancreatitis, Pancreatic carcinoma, Haemochromatosis, Pancreatic resection

Small bowel disease
Coeliac disease, Tropical sprue, Infiltrations *(lymphoma, amyloid, scleroderma)*, Mesenteric vascular insufficiency, Surgical resection

Terminal ileal disease
Regional enteritis, Surgical resection

Bacterial overgrowth
Blind loop, Stricture, Fistula, Decreased gut motility *(amyloid, scleroderma, diabetes mellitus)*

Miscellaneous
Post-gastrectomy, Zollinger-Ellison syndrome, Carcinoid syndrome

Steatorrhoea

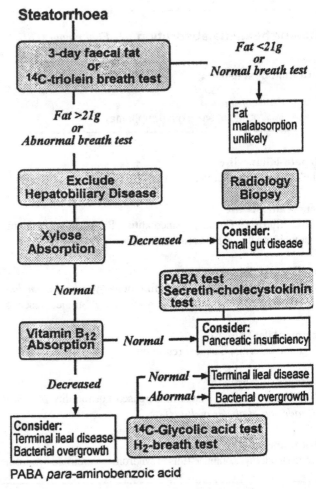

PABA *para*-aminobenzoic acid

Evaluation of steatorrhoea/malabsorption

27 Acute abdominal pain

Acute abdomen *(see Figure page 171)*

> **Laboratory investigations:** play a minor but important role in two areas:
>
> (a) evaluation of the patient's fluid and electrolyte status
> (b) confirmation, or exclusion, of disorders which result in specific biochemical abnormalities, e.g. acute pancreatitis, obstructed bile duct.

(1) Abdominal Causes

Gastrointestinal
Obstruction: Small and large bowel
Perforation: Small and large bowel, peptic ulcer
Infection: Appendicitis, diverticulitis, gastroenteritis

Vascular
Dissecting aneurysm
Ruptured aneurysm
Mesenteric embolus/thrombosis

Pancreas, Hepatobiliary, Spleen
Acute pancreatitis
Acute cholecystitis
Acute cholangitis
Acute hepatitis
Splenic rupture

.... *Cont'd next page*

(abdominal causes cont'd)
Urinary tract
  Urolithiasis
  Acute pyelonephritis

Gynaecological
  Ovary: torsion, ruptured cyst/follicle
  Tubal: Salpingitis, ectopic pregnancy
  Uterus: Endometritis, rupture

---

(2) Acute abdomen: extra-abdominal causes

Endocrine
  Diabetic ketoacidosis
  Addisonian crisis
Haematological
  Acute leukaemia
  Sickle cell crisis
Metabolic
  Acute porphyria
  Uraemia
  Hyperlipoproteinaemia
Drug/Toxins
  Lead toxicity
  Drug withdrawal
Supradiaphram area
  Myocardial infarct
  Pericarditis
  Pulmonary infarct
  Pneumothorax
  Pneumonia

Acute abdominal pain

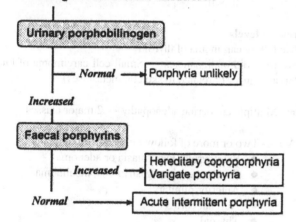

```
Acute abdominal pain
        |
[Clinical Examination]
        |
[Diagnosis uncertain]
        |
Check:
Blood Hb: Haemorrhage
Blood WCC: Infection
Plasma amylase: Acute pancreatitis
                Perforated gut
                Ectopic pregnancy
                Diabetic ketoacidosis
Liver function tests: Hepatobiliary disease
Cardiac enzymes: Myocardial infarct
Plasma glucose: Diabetic ketoacidosis
        |
[Urinary porphobilinogen]
        |
        |— Normal —→ [Porphyria unlikely]
        |
    Increased
        |
[Faecal porphyrins]
        |
        |— Increased —→ [Hereditary coproporphyria
        |                Varigate porphyria]
        |
    Normal ————————→ [Acute intermittent porphyria]
```

Evaluation of abdominal pain

28 Miscellaneous analytes

Tumour markers

> **Tumour markers**
>
> **Definition:** Any substance that can be related to the presence or progress of a tumour.
>
> **Note:** They are of no value and inappropriate for screening the general population for the presence of tumours. Their main value is in monitoring tumour progress.

Calcitonin (CT)

Use: Tumour marker (medullary carcinoma of thyroid). Family screening for MEN II.

Increased levels
- Medullary carcinoma of thyroid
- Non-thyroid malignancies — Small cell carcimoma of lung, Breast cancer (? related to skeletal metastases).

Note: Multiple endocrine adenopathy — 2 major classes

MEN I — Two or more of following glands involved:
- Parathyroid: hyperplasia or adenoma
- Pancreatic islets: gastrinoma, insulinoma
- Anterior pituitary
- Adrenal cortex
- Thyroid

.... *Cont'd next page*

(Multiple endocrine adenosis continued)
MEN II   • Medullary carcinoma of thyroid
            • Phaeochromocytoma
            • Parathyroid hyperplasia or adenoma
            • ± mucocutaneous neurofibroma

Cancer antigen 125 (CA 125)

Uses: Marker for epithelial ovarian carcinoma

Increased levels
- Ovarian tumours (Malignant; Benign, eg endometrioma)
- Non-ovarian malignancy: *Endometrium, Fallopian tubes, Endocervix, Pancreas, Lung, Breast, Colon.*
- Non-malignant disease: *Pregnancy, Menstruation, Endometriosis, Pelvic inflammatory disease, Ovarian hyperstimulation, Adenomyosis, Peritonitis, Acute pancreatitis, Chronic hepatitis, Cirrhosis, Hepatoma.*

Carcinoembryonic antigen (CEA)

Uses: Marker for colorectal malignancy

Increased levels
- Colorectal malignancy
- Non-colorectal malignancy: *Gastric, Lung, Breast, Pancreas*
- Non-malignant diseases: *Inflammatory bowel disease* (gastritis, diverticulitis, ulcerative colitis, Crohn's disease); *Benign liver disease* (hepatitis, cirrhosis, obstructive jaundice, cholestasis); *Pancreatitis; Heavy smokers*

α-Fetoprotein (AFP)

Uses: Marker for hepatocellular carcinoma & germ cell tumours. Asssessment of feotal well being (eg neural tube defects, Trisomy 21, 18 etc)

Increased levels
- Hepatocellular carcinoma
- Germ cell tumours (testes, ovary)
- Non-malignant: *Pregnancy, Liver disease* (Hepatitis) *Hepatocellular regeneration, Ataxic telangiectasia, Hereditary tyrosinaemia*

Human chorionic gonadotropin (β-hCG)

Uses: Tumour marker; monitoring trophoblastic malignancies & germ cell tumours. Detection and monitoring of pregnancy. Antenatal screening for chromosomal abnormalities (triple test).

Increased levels
- Trophoblastic malignancy (choriocarcinoma, hydatidiform mole)
- Non-seminomatous germ cell tumours
- Teratoma
- Pregnancy

Note: (1) Rate of increase or decrease rather than total levels may at times be the more relevant mesurement. (2) When used as tumour marker it is important the β-subunit is estimated.

β₂-Microglobulin

Use: Tumour marker (multiple myeloma). Monitoring renal transplant and glomerular filtration rate...............*Cont'd next page*

(β₂-microglobulin continued)

Increased levels
- Renal impairment (dialysis-dependent, amyloidosis, renal transplant rejection).
- Myeloma, Lymphoma
- AIDS
- SLE, Rheumatoid arthritis, Sarcoidosis

Note: May be of prognostic value in myeloma. Serum levels correlate with tumour cell mass providing there is no renal impairment.

Neuron specific enolase (NSE)

Use: Tumour marker (neuroendocrine tissue, brain, lung)

Increased
- Small cell carcinoma of lung
- Pancreatic islet cell tumours (insulinoma, gastrinoma, etc)
- Medullary carcinoma of thyroid
- Neuroblastoma, Phaeochromocytoma

Note: Haemolysed samples unacceptable for analysis — erythrocytes contain significant amounts of NSE.

Prostate specific antigen (PSA)

Uses: Marker for prostatic malignancy (monitoring therapy and detecting relapses). Forensic marker.

Increased levels
- Prostatic malignancy

.... *Cont'd next page*

(PSA continued)
- Non-malignant disease: *benign prostatic hypertrophy* (3–21% have PSA >10 µg/L), *Prostatitis, Inflammation of other genitourinary tissues, Post-prostatic biopsy.*

Urinary Hydroxymethoxy mandelic acid (HMA, VMA)

Use: Tumour marker for catecholamine producing tumours (phaeochromocytoma, neuroblastoma). Investigation of hypertension.

Increased levels
- Phaeochromocytoma (at least 2-times upper reference level)
- Neuroblastoma (also measure homovanillic acid & dopamine)
- Essential hypertension (mild increase)
- Severe stress (mild to moderate increase)

Note: End product of noradrenaline and adrenaline metabolism. For diagnosis multiple 24-hour collections of urine may be required. MAO inhibitors, L-DOPA, α-methyl dopa, and labetalol will effect results.

Urinary 5-hydroxyindole acetic acid (5-HIAA)

Use: Tumour marker — tumours of argentaffin cells, secreting large amounts of serotonin.

Increased levels
- Carcinoid tumours, especially if metastases to liver (usually >130 µmol/24h)
- Other tumours, eg, oatcell carcinoma of lung
- Small bowel disease — Coeliac disease, Intestinal obstruction

.... *Cont'd next page*

(5-HIAA continued)
- High intake of serotonin containing foods

Note: Multiple collections may be necessary for diagnosis. Before (24h) and during collections avoid fruit and nuts, especially bananas, walnuts, pineapples, plums, avocados and tomatoes.

Angiotensin converting enzyme (ACE)

Uses: Detection and monitoring of sarcoidosis activity. Assessment of ACE inhibition therapy.

Increased levels
- Sarcoidosis
- Other granulomatous disorders (leprosy, tuberculosis)
- Gaucher's disease
- Diabetic microangiopathy
- Hyperthyroidism
- Berylliosis, Silicosis, Asbestosis
- Primary biliary cirrhosis

Decreased levels
- Pulmonary disease (chronic bronchitis, emphysema, malignancy, asthma, cystic fibrosis)
- ACE inhibitory therapy

Note: 40% of subjects with active sarcoidosis have normal serum ACE values.

α_1-Antitrypsin (α_1AT)

Uses: Detection of hereditary α_1AT deficiency. Family screening. Protein-losing enteropathy (faecal measurement)

Decreased levels
- Hereditary α_1AT deficiency

Increased levels
- Inflammation (acute phase reactions)

Note: There are more than 30 genetic variants of this protein. Phenotyping is important & will identify those patients who need to avoid environmental factors that may aggrevate lung damage. Pi ZZ and Pi SS are the most important common variants leading to deficiency. The null variant is uncommon.

Cholinesterase (plasma)

Use: Assessment of cholinesterase inhibitor poisonings, eg organophosphates (malathion). Detection of suxamethonium sensitivity (scoline apnoea); if positive family studies are indicated.

Decreased
- Hepatic damage
- Organophosphate poisoning
- Inherited "abnormal" cholinesterase

Increased
- Nephrotic syndrome
- Recovery from liver damage .... *Cont'd next page*

(Cholinesterase continued)

Note: Use either heparinised plasma or serum — other anticoagulants interfere with the assay.

Caeruloplasmin (plasma)

Use: Diagnosis of Wilson's disease. Assessment of copper metabolism abnormalities.

Decreased
- Wilson's disease (>80% of cases)
- Neonates
- Malnutrition
- Nephrotic syndrome

Increased
- Nonspecific inflammation/malignancy associated with tissue damage
- Third trimester of pregnancy
- Oral contraceptive use
- Active liver disease

C-Reactive Protein (CRP)

Use: Early detection of infection, eg, post-operative, interuterine. Monitoring treatment and disease activity, eg, antibiotic therapy, disease-modifying drugs in rheumatoid arthritis. Assessment of the acute phase response in inflammatory and neoplastic disease.

Increased
- Infection
- Inflammation
- Malignant disease

....*Cont'd next page*

(Increased CRP continued)
- Post-surgical operation

Note: CRP values have been used to differentiate bacterial from viral infections in various clinical situations but this use remains unproven.

Porphyrins/Porphyria

Consider in:
- Unexplained abdominal pain
- Unexplained peripheral neuritis
- Unexplained neurosis or psychosis

Screening tests: *See pages 182, 183 and Table page 181*

- Urine porphyrins (page 182)
- Erythrocyte porphyrins (page 182)
- Porphobilinogen (page 183)

Drugs safe to use in acute porphyria:

Aspirin	Droperidol	Pethidine
Atropine	Ether	Phentanyl
Chlorpromazine	Guanethidine	Propoxyphene
Chloral hydrate	Mefenamic acid	Propranolol
Codeine	Morphine	Phenylbutazone
Corticosteroids	Neostigmine	Rifampicin
Dicoumarol	Nitrous oxide	Succinyldicholine
Dexamethasone	Penicillin	Tetracyclines

Screening & quantitative test results in the porphyrias

| | Screening tests | | | | Quantitative tests | | | | | | | |
| | RBC | Urine | | Faeces | Urine | | | | Faeces | | RBC | |
	Porph	Porph	PBG	Porph	ALA	PBG	Copr	Uro	Copr	Proto	Copr	Proto
Congenital porphyria	✓	✓		✓			✓	✓	✓	✓	✓	✓
Erythropoietic protoporphyria	✓	✓		✓					✓	✓	✓	✓
Acute intermittent porphyria		✓	✓		✓	✓	✓	✓				
Porphyria cutanea tarda		✓ acute attack		✓			✓		✓			
Porphyria variegata		✓ acute attack	✓ acute attack	✓					✓	✓		
Hereditary coproporphyria		✓		✓					✓			
Acquired porphyrinuria		✓			✓		✓	✓				

Porph Porphyrins; PBG Porphobilinogen; ALA δ-amino-laevulinic acid; Copr Coproporphyrinogen;
Uro Uroporphyrinogen; Proto Protoporphyrinogen

Urine porphyrins *(see page 181)*

Use: Screen for suspected porphyria

Increased
- Most porphyrias
- Porphyria cutanea tarda (PCT), in particular
- Lead toxicity

(NOT increased in Erythropoietic protoporphyria)

Erythrocyte porphyrins *(see page 181)*

Use: To diagnose the erythropoietic porphyrias

Increased
- Congenital erythropoietic porphyria
- Erythropoietic protoporphyria
- Any condition with impaired red cell development (eg, lead toxicity, iron deficient anaemia)

Faecal porphyrins *(see page 181)*

Use: Diagnosis of acute porphyria

Increased
- Erythropoietic protoporphyria
- Porphyria variegata
- Hereditary coproporphyria

(In PCT isocoproporphyrin fraction increased)

Urine porphobilinogen (PBG) *(see page 181)*

Use: Screen for acute porphyria

Increased
- Acute intermittent porphyria (AIP)
- Hereditary coproporphyria
- Porphyria variegata

(NOTE PBG not increased during latent phases though increase may persist in AIP despite clinical recovery)

Cerebrospinal fluid (CSF)

Appearance

Red: Suggests recent haemorrhage into subarachnoid space or lumbar puncture trauma

Yellow: (Xanthrochromia)
- Altered haemoglobin
- Increased white blood cells
- Increased protein content:
  Cervical/spinal tumour,
  infection, Post seizure,
  Neonates and infants

Turbid: Excess white or red blood cells

Biochemistry

A. Glucose (value rarely less than 50% of plasma level)

.... *Cont'd next page*

(CSF glucose continued)
Low glucose
- Infection, especially bacterial including TB (cannot distinguish between different forms of infective meningitis)
- Hypoglycaemia
- Widespread malignant infiltration of meninges

B. Protein

Increased total protein
- Blood
- White blood cells
- Non-purulent inflammation of CNS
- Spinal canal blockage
- Post seizure
- Neonates and infants

Specific proteins
- CSF electrophoresis compared with serum electrophoresis may provide answers to specific questions
- CSF normally has a higher pre-albumin level & lower γ-globulin level (re serum)
- When there is a breakdown of the blood-brain barrier higher molecular weight proteins may be detected in the CSF (ie not normally present in large amounts). *Consider: Multiple sclerosis, Cerebral tumours, Encephalitis, Neurosyphilis, SLE, Guillian-Barre' syndrome, Cerebral sarcoidosis, Slow viral disease, Subacute sclerosing pan encephalitis*
- (?) Rhinorrhoea/Otorrhoea OR (?) CSF: Send sample with corresponding serum to laboratory for Tau band demonstration (Tau band of CSF is formed from transferrin degradation products).

29 Dynamic function tests

Ammonium chloride loading/urinary acidification

Aim: To test ability of distal renal tubules to acidify urine

Use: Confirmation of diagnosis of renal tubular acidosis

Patient preparation: No food or fluid to be taken after midnight

Dose: 0.1 g/kg NH_4Cl orally (gelatin capsule) at 08.00 h.

Samples: Empty bladder (discard) at 08.00 h prior to dose

1. Collect urine specimens hourly until 16.00 h
2. Specimens to laboratory for estimation of pH, titratable acidity
   & ammonia

Interpretation: See Table page 43.

Normal: pH <5.50, titratable acidity >25µmol/min, ammonia >35 µmol/min.

Type 1 RTA: pH >5.50, titratable acidity <25µmol/min, ammonia <35 µmol/min.

Type 2 RTA: pH <5.50, titratable acidity >25µmol/min, ammonia >35 µmol/min.

Type 4 RTA: pH <5.50, titratable acidity >25µmol/min, ammonia <35 µmol/min.

Aldosterone/Renin: Postural response

Aim: To test ability of aldosterone-renin axis to respond to postural changes.

Use: Evaluation of mineralocorticoid deficiency syndromes

Patient preparation: Nil specific. Stope diuretics for at least one week prior to test.

Protocol: Blood specimens for aldosterone and plasma renin activity (PRA) are taken:

1. Prior to getting out of bed in the morning
2. After 3 h ambulation

Interpretation:

Normal: At least a two-fold increase in both aldosterone and PRA

No response to ambulation (decreased PRA & aldosterone)
    Syndrome of hyporeninaemic hypoaldosteronism
    Prostaglandin inhibitors
PRA high but no aldosterone response to ambulation
    Aldosterone synthesis defect
    Captopril therapy
    Heparin therapy
Recumbent PRA & aldosterone both high
    Tubule unresponsiveness to aldosterone

Plasma aldosterone response to salt load

Aim: To test autonomy of aldosterone secretion

Use: Evaluation of suspected primary hyperaldosteronism

Patient preparation: Stop all medications (inc. Diuretics) for at least one week prior to test.

Protocol: Two methods

1. High salt diet (15--250 mmol/day) for one week

2. Infuse 2 L of normal saline at 500 mL/h over 4 h.

Blood sample for plasma aldosterone taken before and after salt load.

Interpretation:

Normal: Plasma aldosterone suppresses to below 240 pmol/L

Primary hyperaldosteronism: No suppression or Plasma aldosterone remains above 420 pmol/L.

Synacthen stimulation

Aim: Evaluation of adrenal cortex reserve

Use: Evaluation of possible adrenal hypofunction

Short Synacthen Test

Use: Screen for adrenal insufficiency

Patient preparation: perform at 09.00 h if possible

Dose: 250 mg Synacthen by IM injection

Blood samples: Basal, 30 min, & 60 min for plasma cortisol

Interpretation:

Normal response: Both of following in one or both post-stimulation samples.

1. Basal value exceeded by at least 200 nmol/L
2. An absolute level of 550 nmol/L exceeded.

Complete failure to respond: primary adrenal failure

Partial or sluggish response (criteria not fulfilled & 60 min value >30 min value): Possible secondary hypoadrenalism - proceed to prolonged stimulation.

.... *Cont'd next page*

Prolonged Synacthen test

Use: Evaluate an inadequate response to the short test

Dose: 1 mg Depot Synacthen IM

Blood samples: Basal, 0.5, 1, 1.5, 2, 4, 6, 8, 12, 24 h (for plasma cortisol)

Interpretation:

Normal response: Short Synacthen criteria met by 1 hour sample
Primary Addison's disease: No significant rise
Pituitary disease: Delayed slow rise reaching a maximum at 24h

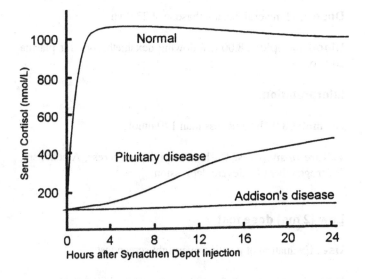

Plasma cortisol response to Depot Synacthen

Dexamethasone suppression tests

Aim: Investigate negative feedback mechanism of hypothalamic-pituitary-adrenal axis.

Use: Evaluation of suspected hypercortisolism

Overnight test

Use: Screening for inappropriate hypercortisolism

Patient preparation: Nil

Dose: 1–2 mg oral dexamethasone at 23.00 h

Blood sample: 08.00 h following dexamethasone for plasma cortisol

Interpretation:

Normal: 08.00 h value less than 140 nmol/L

Failure to suppress: Cushing's syndrome, Stress, Alcoholism, Oestrogen therapy, Severe depression

Low (2 mg) dose test

Use: Evaluation of positive overnight screen test

Dose: 0.5 mg 6-hourly for 48 h (commence 07.00 day 1)

(Low dose dexamethasone continued)

Blood samples: 07.00 on day 3 for plasma cortisol estimation

Interpretation: As for the overnight test

High (8 mg) dose test

Use: Determine aetiology of Cushing's syndrome

Dose: 2 mg orally 6-hourly for 48 hours (commence 07.00 h on day 1)

Blood samples: 07.00 h on day 3

Interpretation:

1. Suppression of the day 3 plasma cortisol to less than 50% of the basal level occurs in pituitary-dependent Cushing's disease

2. Failure to suppress occurs in:

   • Adrenal tumours
   • Ectopic-ACTH syndrome

NB Adrenal tumours may secrete cortisol intermittently and thus produce a false suppression in the above tests

Thyrotropin-releasing hormone (TRH) Stimulation

Aim: To assess
1. anterior pituitary reserve of TSH
2. level of negative feedback by plasma thyroid hormones

Use: *Hypothyroidism:* Evaluate possible secondary disease
Hyperthyroidism: Diagnosis when plasma tests equivocal

Patient preparation: Nil

TRH dose: 200 mg given IV

Blood samples: Basal, 20, 60 min post dose for plasma TSH

Interpretation:

Normal response: At least 3-fold increase in plasma TSH with 20 min value exceeding 60 min value (some consider an increase of >2.0 mIU/L as normal).

Inadequate response:

(1) No increase in conjunction with (a) depressed serum free thyroxine level and (b) a basal TSH below upper reference limit is suggestive of inadequate pituitary reserve. A sluggish response with the 60 min value greater than the 20 min value suggests hypothalamic disease.

(2) No TSH response in association with an elevated serum free thyroxine or serum tri-iodothyronine, or both strongly suggests thyrotoxicosis.

Triple function test

Aim: To evaluate anterior pituitary reserve of hormones

Use: Evaluate suspected hypopituitarism

Patient preparation: Must be performed under medical supervision and a 50% glucose solution should be available for IV injection. *Contra indications:* cardiac & cerebrovascular disease.

Dose: For adults

Insulin (soluble): 0.05–0.15 units/kg body wt
TRH: 200 μg
GnRH: 100 μg

Given IV as a bolus dose

> Clinical signs and symptoms of hypoglycaemia (sweating, tachycardia, etc) indicate adequate stress (plasma glucose usually falls to below 2.8 mmol/L) If signs of severe hypoglycaemia IV glucose should be given and the test terminated.

Blood samples: Basal, 30, 60, 90, 120 min for plasma Glucose, Cortisol, GH, LH, FSH, TSH, Prolactin

NB If doubt regarding adrenocortical function a short Synacthen test (page 188) should be performed following the final blood sampling.

.... *Cont'd next page*

(triple function test continued)

Interpretation: *Normal response:*

Cortisol - Rise to above 200 nmol/L
GH - Rise to at least 20 mU/L
TSH - At least a 3-fold rise
Prolactin - Greater than 10-fold rise
LH - Greater than 5-fold rise
FSH - Greater than 3-fold rise

The responses of the various hormones will indicate the pituitary reserve of each, ie, no response - complete loss, partial response - partial loss, etc

---

Growth hormone stimulation test

Aim: Evaluate pituitary reserve of GH

Exercise Test

Use: Screening test for GH deficiency in children

Patient preparation: perform at least 3 h after last meal

Exercise: Workload appropriate for subject's size on a bicycle ergometer, or stair-running for 20-30 min.

Blood samples: Basal, 1, 2, 20 min after cessation of exercise for Plasma GH

Interpretation: Normal response if plasma GH exceeds 20 mU/L.

L-Dopa stimulation

Use: Test for GH deficiency in children

Patient preparation: Patient supine during test

Dose: Oral levodopa: >30 kg 500 mg; 15–30 kg 250 mg; <15 kg 125 mg

Blood samples: Basal, 30, 60, 90 for Plasma GH

Interpretation: Normal response if plasma GH exceeds 20 mU/L.

Growth hormone suppression test

Oral glucose tolerance test

Aim: Evaluate suppressibility of circulating GH

Patient preparation & protocol : As for OGTT on page 196.

Blood samples: Basal, 30, 60, 90, 120 for glucose & GH

Interpretation:

A normal response occurs if at least one GH value falls to below 1 mU/L. In acromegaly there is little or no suppression.

Oral glucose tolerance test (OGTT)

Use: 1. Evaluate glucose tolerance in subjects with equivocal
features of diabetes mellitus and do not have fasting
blood glucose values in excess of 7.8 mmol/L
2. Suppression of growth hormone secretion in patients
with suspected acromegaly

Patient preparation: Essential to standardise the test.

♦ Normal diet & carbohydrate intake (>150 g/d) for 3 days
♦ Overnight fast (10–16 hours)
♦ Resting for 30 min (seated) prior to test
♦ No smoking during test
♦ No drugs known to interfere with test, eg, steroids

Glucose load: Adult 75 g; children 1.75 g/kg (max. of 75 g)

Protocol:

Must be performed in morning and to remain seated (no exercise)
during test.

Glucose load given in flavoured water and consumed within 5 min.

Urine glucose estimations are not essential during test but useful if
renal glycosuria a possibility.

Blood samples: Basal (pre-glucose), 60 min, 120 min (into
tubes containing sodium fluoride)

.... *Cont'd next page*

(OGTT continued)

Interpretation:

Normal

Basal	<6.4	mmol/L
Intermediate sample	<11.1	mmol/L
2 h sample	<7.8	mmol/L

Diabetic
Basal	Variable	
Intermediate sample	<11.1	mmol/L
2 h sample	>11.1	mmol/L

Impaired glucose tolerance

Basal	<7.8	mmol/L
Intermediate sample	variable	
2 h sample	7.8–11.1	mmol/L

Non-diagnostic

Any response that does not fulfil the above criteria.

Dehydration - Renal concentration test

Aim: Determine integrity of hypothalamic-pituitary-renal urinary concentrating apparatus.

Use: Evaluation of polyuria

Patient preparation: No fluid or food after 9 PM
the night before the test   ....*Cont'd next page*

(dehydration test continued)

Protocol:

Subject must not take fluids during test
Weigh subject hourly and abort test if weight falls by 5%.

1. Estimate osmolality on early morning urine:

   If >800 mmol/L terminate test as patient normal
   If <800 mmol/kg proceed to 2.

2. Beginning as early as possible in morning (eg, 07.00 h) empty
   bladder completely & estimate osmolality on the sample.

3. Perform this exercise every 60 min until:

   (A) Urine osmoality exceeds 800 mmol/Kg (normal) **OR**
   (B) Urinary osmolality reaches a plateau (consecutive
       osmolalities agree with in 30 mmol/kg)

4. When urinary osmolality plateau reached:

   a. Take blood for plasma osmolality estimation
   b. Administer arginine vasopressin (5 units SC or equivalent by
      nasal spray)

5. Take a final urine sample 60 min after AVP administration

Interpretation: (see Figure page 162)

Normal response: Urine osmolality rises to beyond 800 mmol/kg
without exogenous AVP stimulation.

.... *Cont'd next page*

(interpretation of dehydration test continued)

Neurogenic diabetes insipidus: Urinary osmolality does not rise beyond 300 mmol/kg. Following AVP administration there is a rapid increase in urinary osmolality to above 800 mmol/kg (or increase by >70% over basal level).

Partial neurogenic diabetes insipidus: Pre-AVP urine osmolality >300 mmol/kg but <800 mmol/kg. Post-AVP urine osmolality >800 mmol/kg.

Nephrogenic diabetes insipidus: urine osmolality does not rise beyond 300 mmol/kg and no response to exogenous AVP.

Partial nephrogenic diabetes insipidus: Pre-AVP urine 300–800 mmol/kg and no response post-AVP.

Notes on concentration test

Anomalous results

♦ Surreptitious drinking during test
♦ Contamination with residual (dilute) urine

Polyuria due to overdrinking

These subjects may show a partial nephrogenic response due to wash-out of osmotic particles during a long period of diuresis.

Glossary of Abbreviations

[x]	Concentration of x	AVP	Arginine vasopressin (antidiuretic hormone, ADH)
↑	Increase		
↑↑	Large increase		
↓	Decrease	Bili	Bilirubins
↓↓	Large decrease	BJP	Bence-Jones protein
~	Approximately	Ca^{2+}	Calcium ion
		Ca	Calcium
AcAc	Acetoacetic acid	CAT	Computerized axial tomography
ACE	Angiotensin-converting enzyme		
ACP	Acid phosphatase	CBG	Cortisol-binding globulin
ACTH	Adrenocorticotrophic hormone (corticotrophin)	CCF	Congestive cardiac failure
		CEA	Carcinoembryonic antigen
ADH	Antidiuretic hormone (arginine vasopressin, AVP)	Chol	Cholesterol
		CK	Creatine kinase
αFP	α-Fetoprotein	Cl	Chloride
Agap	Anion gap	Cl^-	Chloride ion
AIP	Acute intermittent porphyria	CNS	Central nervous system
Alb	Albumin	COAD	Chronic obstructive airways disease, Ephysema
Aldo	Aldosterone		
ALP	Alkaline phosphatase		
ALT	Alanine aminotransferase	Cort	Cortisol
		Creat	Creatinine
AMI	Acute myocardial infarction	CRF	Chronic renal failure
		CSF	Cerebrospinal fluid
Amy	Amylase	DHCC	Dihydroxycholecalciferol
ARF	Acute renal failure		
AST	Aspartate amino transferase	DHEAS	Dehydroepiandrosterone sulphate
ATN	Acute tubular necrosis	DHT	Dihydrotestosterone

E₂	Oestradiol	**Hb**	Haemoglobin
ECF	Extracellular fluid	**HBD**	Hydroxybutyrate
ECV	Extracellular volume		dehydrogenase
EDTA	Ethylenediamine tetra-	**HCMA**	Hyperchloraemic
	acetate (sequestrene)		metabolic acidosis
EIA	Electro-immunoassay	**HCO₃**	Bicarbonate
ELISA	Enzyme-linked	**HCO₃⁻**	Bicarbonate ion
	immunosorbant assay	**HDL**	High density lipo-
ESR	Erythrocyte sedimen-		proteins
	tation rate	**Hg**	Mercury
		5HT	5-Hydroxytryptamine
Fe	Iron	**5HIAA**	5-hydroxyindone
Fex	Fractional excretion of		acetic acid
	x	**HMMA**	4-Hydroxy-3-methoxy-
αFP	α-Fetoprotein		mandelic acid (VMA)
FSH	Follicle-stimulating	**HVA**	Homovanillic acid
	hormone		
fT₃	Free triiodothyronine	**IDDM**	Insulin-dependent
fT₄	Free thyroxine		diabetes mellitus
FTI	Free thyroxine index	**IHD**	Ischaemic heart
			disease
GFR	Glomerular filtration	**IM**	Intramuscular
	rate	**IV**	Intravenous
GF	Glomerular filtrate	**IVV**	Intravascular volume
GGT	Gamma-glutamyl-		
	transferase	**K**	Potassium
GH	Growth hormone	**K⁺**	Potassium ion
GHRF	Growth hormone		
	releasing factor	**LD**	Lactate dehydrog-
Glob	Globulins		enase
Glu	Glucose	**LDL**	Low density lipo-
GnRH	Gonadotrophin-		proteins
	releasing hormone	**LFT**	Liver function tests
GTT	Glucose tolerance	**LH**	Luteinizing hormone
	test	**LHRH**	Luteinizing hormone-
			releasing hormone
H⁺	Hydrogen ion		
HAGMA	High anion gap	**MEA**	Multiple endocrine
	metabolic acidosis		adenoma

MEN Multiple endocrine
neoplasia
Mg Magnesium
Mg^{2+} Magnesium ion
MI Myocardial infarction

Na Sodium
Na$^+$ Sodium ions
NAGMA Normal anion gap
metabolic acidosis
NIDDM Non-insulin depen-
dent diabetes
mellitus
5'-NT 5'-Nucleotidase

β-OHB β-hydroxybutyric acid
Osmol Osmolality

P$_1$ Progesterone
PA Plasma aldosterone
PBG Porphobilinogen
PCOD Polycystic ovarian
disease
Pco$_2$ Partial pressure of
carbon dioxide
Po$_2$ Partial pressure of
oxygen
PO$_4$ Inorganic phosphate
PRA Plasma renin activity
PRL Prolactin
PRU Pre-renal uraemia
PTH Parathyroid hormone
PTHrP PTH-related protein

RIA Radioimmunoassay
RR Referenc range
RTA Renal tubular acidosis

SD Standard deviation
SHBG Sex hormone-
binding globulin
SHH Syndrome of hypo-
reninaemic hypo-
aldosteronism
SIADH Syndrome of inappropriate secretion of
ADH

T$_3$ Triiodothyronine
T$_4$ Thyroxine
Te Testosterone
tT$_3$ Total triiodothyronine
tT$_4$ Total thyroxine
TA Titratable acidity
TBG Thyroxine-binding
globulins
TBP Thyroxine-binding
proteins
Te Testosterone
TIBC Total iron binding
capacity
TProt Total protein
TSH Thyroid-stimulating
hormone (thyro-
trophin)
TRH Thyrotorphin-
releasing hormone
Trig Triglycerides

Uosmol Urine osmolality
VLDL Very low density
lipoproteins
VMA Vanillyl mandelic acid

Index